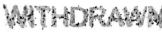
# Fast Facts:
# Prostate Cancer

## Ninth edition

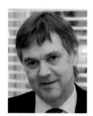

**Roger S Kirby** MA MD FRCS(Urol) FEBU
Professor of Urology
The Prostate Centre
London, UK

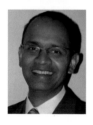

**Manish I Patel** MBBS MMED PhD FRACS
Associate Professor, University of Sydney
Urological Cancer Surgeon
Westmead Hospital
Sydney, Australia

**Declaration of Independence**
This book is as balanced and as practical as we can make it.
Ideas for improvement are always welcome: feedback@fastfacts.com

D1422207

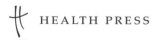

HEALTH PRESS

Fast Facts: Prostate Cancer
First published 1996; second edition 1998; third edition 2001; fourth edition 2004;
fifth edition 2008; sixth edition 2009; seventh edition 2012; eighth edition 2014
Ninth edition March 2017; reprinted July 2017

Text © 2017 Roger S Kirby, Manish I Patel
© 2017 in this edition Health Press Limited

Health Press Limited, Elizabeth House, Queen Street, Abingdon,
Oxford OX14 3LN, UK
Tel: +44 (0)1235 523233

Book orders can be placed by telephone or via the website.
To order via the website, please go to: fastfacts.com
For telephone orders, please call +44 (0)1752 202301

Fast Facts is a trademark of Health Press Limited.

A CIP record for this title is available from the British Library.

ISBN 978-1-910797-37-2

Kirby RS (Roger)
Fast Facts: Prostate Cancer/
Roger S Kirby, Manish I Patel

Medical illustrations by Dee McLean, London, UK, and
Annamaria Dutto, Beverley, UK.
Typesetting by Thomas Bohm, User Design, Illustration and Typesetting, UK.
Printed in the UK with Xpedient Print.

# Glossary of abbreviations

**ADT:** androgen deprivation therapy

**AUA:** American Urological Association

**BMD:** bone mineral density

**BPH:** benign prostatic hyperplasia

**CRPC:** castrate-resistant prostate cancer

**CT:** computed tomography

**CYP17:** cytochrome P450 17-hydroxylase/17,20-lyase

**DES:** diethylstilbestrol

**DHT:** dihydrotestosterone

**DRE:** digital rectal exam

**EBRT:** external-beam radiotherapy

**HDL:** high-density lipoprotein

**HIFU:** high-intensity focused ultrasonography

**IMRT:** intensity-modulated radiotherapy

**LDL:** low-density lipoprotein

**LH:** luteinizing hormone

**LHRH:** luteinizing hormone-releasing hormone

**mpMRI:** multiparametric magnetic resonance imaging

**NNT:** number needed to treat (to save one death)

**OS:** overall survival

**PDE:** phosphodiesterase

**PET:** positron emission tomography

**PSA:** prostate-specific antigen

**PSMA:** prostate-specific membrane antigen

**RANKL:** receptor activator of nuclear factor κB ligand

**TNM:** tumor–nodes–metastasis (staging system)

**TRUS:** transrectal ultrasonography

**TURP:** transurethral resection of the prostate

**USPSTF:** US Preventive Services Task Force

**VTP:** vascular-targeted photodynamic therapy

# Introduction

Prostate cancer is unusual among solid tumors in that many men die *with*, rather than *of*, the disease – the lifetime risk of developing clinical prostate cancer in western countries is about 1 in 8, but many cancers grow slowly, such that the risk of developing clinically detectable cancer is about 13%, and the lifetime risk of actually dying from prostate cancer is approximately 3%. This raises many challenges for both healthcare professionals and patients in terms of deciding *if*, *when* and *how* to intervene in order to control tumor growth and spread, thereby extending survival but without compromising quality of life. Survivorship is therefore an important issue, and is discussed in Chapter 9.

This is the ninth edition of this *Fast Facts* handbook since the first was published in 1996, testament to the rapid changes in the field and steadily improving outlook for patients. This new edition introduces the Gleason grade grouping (Chapter 1), which has valuable prognostic value, and nomograms that are used to evaluate risk (Chapter 4). Our understanding of the genetics and underlying pathogenesis of prostate cancer is growing apace, leading to the identification of germline mutations and the development of genomic tests to help identify those at greatest risk of developing clinically significant disease (Chapter 3). Imaging techniques are also improving rapidly, particularly multiparametric MRI (Chapter 4), and, by identifying specific target areas, are improving the accuracy of the biopsy process and reducing the number of negative biopsies.

The androgen receptor is central to the pathogenesis of prostate cancer – rather like the estrogen receptor in breast cancer – and manipulation of the hormone milieu is key in treatment; however, androgen deprivation has considerable effect on quality of life, prompting continued exploration of the optimal timing and sequencing of treatment, including the concept of intermittent androgen blockade (Chapters 7 and 8).

Methods for detecting and monitoring the disease are also improving. The role of prostate-specific antigen (PSA) in the screening, detection and monitoring of prostate cancer and its treatment is persistently controversial, with advocates for and against. Nevertheless, measurement of serum PSA continues to provide valuable information to inform clinical decisions, although it is hoped that other markers, whether complimentary or as an alternative, will emerge with time. Different measures of PSA, such as the doubling time and velocity are being explored; the Prostate Health Index is a combined measure, approved in the USA (Chapter 3).

The debate over the merits of surgery versus radiotherapy for patients with localized but high-risk disease continues, especially as robot-assisted surgery, low-dose seed brachytherapy and CyberKnife targeted radiation therapy continue to improve accuracy and precision (Chapter 5). Chemotherapy with docetaxel at initiation of androgen-ablation therapy has become the standard of care for men with metastatic prostate cancer, and either enzalutamide or abiraterone for men with castrate-resistant prostate cancer (CRPC). Immunotherapies and vaccines are now also being explored, and offer further hope to men with CRPC (Chapter 8).

With this ninth edition of this popular *Fast Facts* handbook, we hope to help those who provide support and care for men with prostate cancer to feel fully informed in navigating the complexities of clinical decision-making. Because the book is concise, fully up to date and evidence based, we believe it is an ideal resource for primary care providers, specialist nurses, trainee urologists and allied healthcare professionals, who want to get quickly up to speed in this fast-moving field. You can swiftly test your knowledge after reading this book by taking our FastTest at fastfacts.com, and please do post a comment for us on the site if you have any specific feedback.

Prostate cancer is the most common malignancy to affect men of middle age and beyond in most developed countries and, increasingly in developing countries, it is second only to lung cancer as a cause of cancer deaths in men. The lifetime risk of developing clinical prostate cancer in western countries is about 1 in 8. Approximately 80% of men aged 80 years have prostate cancer at autopsy. However, many of these cancers grow slowly and the risk of developing clinically detectable cancer is about 13%; the lifetime risk of actually dying from prostate cancer is approximately 3%.

Worldwide, there has been a steady increase in the incidence of clinically significant prostate cancer, although in the USA the number of incidental diagnoses of prostate cancer has fallen by 28% since the US Preventive Task Force issued a draft guideline in 2011 (which became a final recommendation 2012) discouraging prostate-specific antigen (PSA)-based screening in all men (Figure 1.1).

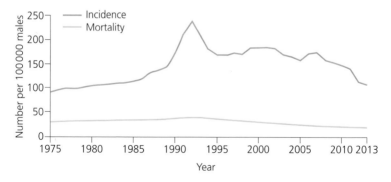

**Figure 1.1** The incidence and mortality of prostate cancer in the USA from 1975 to 2013. The temporary rise in incidence coincides with the introduction of PSA screening in about 1990, although the US Preventive Services Task Force guidelines issued in 2011/12 now discourage screening in all men. Data are from the US National Cancer Institute (NCI) Surveillance Epidemiology and End Results (SEER; https://seer.cancer.gov/statfacts/html/prost.html, last accessed 07 March 2017).

However, prostate cancer primarily affects men over the age of 50 years, so the number of men diagnosed with prostate cancer is predicted to increase substantially over the next two decades as a result of the worldwide trend towards an aging population. The debate around measurement of PSA is discussed in detail in Chapter 3 (pages 36–9).

Mortality from prostate cancer in Europe rose to a peak in 1993, reached a plateau, and has now started to decrease. Mortality in the USA has also shown similar trends (see Figure 1.1); the rate of decline has increased significantly in recent years and is now four times faster than in the UK. Some have attributed this drop to the efforts made in North America to detect and treat prostate cancer early through PSA testing a decade or two earlier, although several other factors may also have contributed, such as changes in lifestyle and better treatment outcomes.

## Risk factors

Despite the high incidence of prostate cancer, relatively little is known about the underlying causes. However, several risk factors have been identified (Table 1.1).

**Age** is the greatest factor that influences the development of prostate cancer. Clinical disease is rare in men under the age of 50 years but the incidence increases markedly over 60 years of age.

**Race.** Marked geographic and racial variations are seen in the incidence of clinical prostate cancer (Table 1.2). The risk is highest in

TABLE 1.1

**Established and possible risk factors for prostate cancer**

- Aging
- Race
- Family history
- Hormones
- Genetic polymorphism
- Obesity
- Western-style diet
- Low exposure to sunlight

TABLE 1.2

**Incidence of prostate cancer according to race in the USA**

| Ethnicity | Number of cases (per 100 000) |
|---|---|
| All races | 20.7 |
| Black | 44.2 |
| Non-Hispanic | 20.9 |
| White | 19.1 |
| American Indian/Alaskan native | 19.1 |
| Hispanic | 17.1 |
| Asian/Pacific islander | 9.1 |

Source: SEER Stat Fact Sheets: Prostate Cancer https://seer.cancer.gov/statfacts/html/prost.html, last accessed 07 March 2017.

North America and northern European countries, and lowest in the Far East. In the USA, the risk is higher in black men than in white men, and black men also appear to develop more aggressive disease earlier. The incidence of prostate cancer is lowest in Chinese and Japanese races, although the prevalence is now increasing in both. The incidence of latent (clinically insignificant) disease is similar in all populations studied. The incidence of prostate cancer in men who emigrate from a low- to a high-risk area increases to that of the local population within two generations. This suggests that environmental influences such as diet and lifestyle factors may have a profound effect on the development of prostate cancer and on the progression of latent to clinically detectable cancer.

**Family history/genetic risk.** Epidemiology studies show that heritable factors account for a small proportion of prostate cancer risk but a higher proportion of early-onset disease. However, a host of studies have suggested the existence of prostate cancer susceptibility genes. Family history is a strong risk factor for prostate cancer: the risk of a man developing prostate cancer is increased approximately 2.5-fold if he has a first-degree relative who is affected. The relative risks for developing prostate cancer based on family history are shown in Table 1.3.

TABLE 1.3

**Risk of developing prostate cancer in relation to family history of the disease**

| Relative | Age at diagnosis | Relative risk (95% confidence interval) |
|---|---|---|
| ≥ 2 first-degree | Any | 4.39 (2.61, 7.39) |
| Brother(s) | Any | 3.14 (2.37, 4.15) |
| First-degree | < 65 years | 2.87 (2.21, 3.74) |
| Second-degree | Any | 2.52 (0.99, 6.46) |
| First-degree | Any | 2.48 (2.25, 2.74) |
| Father | Any | 2.35 (2.02, 2.72) |
| First-degree relative | ≥ 65 years | 1.92 (1.49, 2.47) |

Adapted from Kiciński M et al. *PLoS One* 2011;6:e27130.

The high incidence of familial prostate cancer prompted a search for germline mutations. Early linkage analyses suggested the human prostate cancer 1 gene (*HPC1*) located at 1q24–25, and studies in men with familial prostate cancer but without male to male transmission led to the identification of the X-linked human prostate cancer X gene (*HPCX*) at Xq27–28. Further loci have also been identified on chromosomes 2, 3, 5, 6, 8, 10, 11, 13, 15, 17, 19, 20 and 22. Familial prostate cancer is a far more heterogenous condition than familial breast cancer, with contributions from many more gene loci. The predictive value of any one allele is low; hence, a clinically useful genetic test has not yet been identified.

The strongest evidence for direct causality comes from families who develop cancer syndromes such as Lynch syndrome – the risk of developing prostate cancer is elevated twofold for those carrying the abnormal gene.

Mutations in the *BRCA2* breast cancer susceptibility gene are rare in men with prostate cancer but appear to be associated with earlier diagnosis and more aggressive disease, such as higher Gleason score (see pages 14–16) and higher PSA level and tumor stage and/or grade at diagnosis. Furthermore, carriers of *BRCA2* mutations may have lower overall survival (OS) and prostate cancer-specific survival compared with non-carriers. Knowledge of a man's *BRCA2* status therefore has prognostic value. The US National Cancer Institute web pages on the genetics of prostate cancer provide a thorough review of the current status of this fast-changing field and are updated regularly (www.cancer.gov/types/prostate/hp/prostate-genetics-pdq).

**Hormones.** Testosterone and its more potent metabolite dihydrotestosterone (DHT) are essential for normal prostate growth and also play a role in the development of prostate cancer (Figure 1.2). Prostate cancer almost never develops in the rare case of men who are for some reason castrated before puberty, or in men deficient in 5α-reductase – the enzyme with type I and II isoforms that converts testosterone to DHT. Trials have shown that the type II 5α-reductase inhibitors finasteride and dutasteride reduce the development of prostate cancer by about 25%, suggesting a key role for DHT. However, the incidence of prostate cancer increases with age, while serum testosterone levels decrease. In addition, men diagnosed with advanced prostate cancer often have a lower average testosterone level than men of a similar age who do not have prostate cancer.

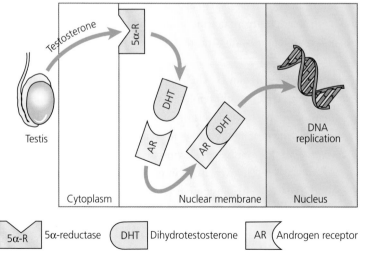

**Figure 1.2** Testosterone, which is converted to DHT by 5α-reductase, supports prostate cell function and stimulates cell division.

**Obesity.** Early studies showed an increased risk of prostate cancer in obese men whereas more recent studies indicate that levels of detected prostate cancer are in fact lower in obese men. This may be because they have lower levels of PSA and androgens, such that fewer obese men underwent biopsy and were diagnosed with prostate cancer in the PSA era. A recently published study on risk factors for prostate cancer reported that being obese was associated with a 44% increase in the risk of prostate cancer diagnosis. Prostate cancer mortality is significantly higher in men who are obese. The mechanism by which obesity increases the likelihood of death from prostate cancer is not known but may be through the activation of pro-carcinogenic pathways such as the insulin-like growth factor (IGF) axis.

**Western diets** tend to be high in animal fat, protein, meat and processed carbohydrates, and low in plant foods. A number of studies support links between the intake of saturated fat and red and processed meats in particular and the development of prostate cancer. There is also some evidence that α-linoleic acid, an omega-3 polyunsaturated fatty acid, increases the risk of prostate cancer and of developing advanced disease, which may be the result of oxidative stress and subsequent DNA damage or the development of obesity. Omega-3 fatty acids from marine sources may, however, decrease the risk of developing prostate cancer.

**Sun exposure and vitamin D.** The risk of dying from prostate cancer is related geographically to ultraviolet (UV) light exposure, and men with prostate cancer have lower levels of vitamin D. Vitamin D levels are determined by dietary intake and conversion in the skin by UV light; however, the mechanism by which vitamin D levels protect against prostate cancer is not known, and vitamin D supplementation doe not decrease the risk. Calcitriol (vitamin D) has been used in the treatment of advanced prostate cancer but evidence of efficacy is lacking.

### Histological features

Most prostate cancers are adenocarcinomas. The majority (>70%) appear to arise in the peripheral zone of the gland (Figure 1.3); 5–15%

arise in the central zone and the remainder from the transition zone, which is where benign prostatic hyperplasia (BPH) also develops.

Microscopic foci of 'latent' prostate cancer are a common autopsy finding and may appear very early in life: approximately 30% of men over 50 years of age have evidence of latent disease. However, these microscopic tumors often grow very slowly, and many never progress to clinical disease. Beyond a certain size, however, these lesions progressively de-differentiate, probably as a result of clonal selection, and become increasingly invasive. A tumor with a volume greater than

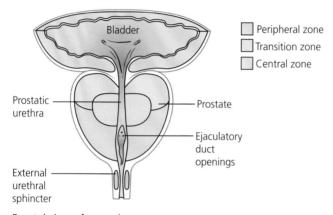

Peripheral zone
Transition zone
Central zone

Bladder

Prostatic urethra

Prostate

Ejaculatory duct openings

External urethral sphincter

Frontal view of normal prostate

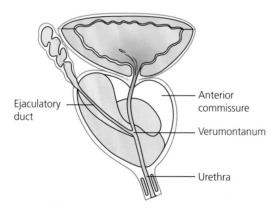

Ejaculatory duct

Anterior commissure

Verumontanum

Urethra

Sagittal view of normal prostate

**Figure 1.3** Approximately 70% of prostate cancers arise in the peripheral zone.

0.5 cm$^3$ or that is anything other than well differentiated is generally regarded as clinically significant.

**The Gleason grading system** is widely used for grading prostate cancer (Figure 1.4). In this system, the tumor is first graded 1–5 according to aggressiveness; the numbers of the two most widely represented grades

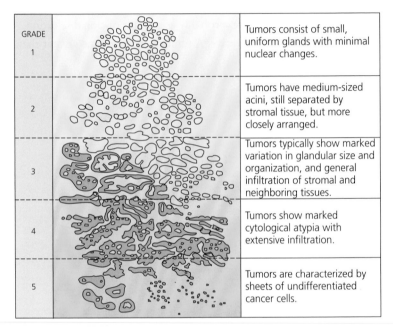

| GRADE 1 | | Tumors consist of small, uniform glands with minimal nuclear changes. |
| GRADE 2 | | Tumors have medium-sized acini, still separated by stromal tissue, but more closely arranged. |
| GRADE 3 | | Tumors typically show marked variation in glandular size and organization, and general infiltration of stromal and neighboring tissues. |
| GRADE 4 | | Tumors show marked cytological atypia with extensive infiltration. |
| GRADE 5 | | Tumors are characterized by sheets of undifferentiated cancer cells. |

**Figure 1.4** The Gleason grading system is based on the extent to which the tumor cells are arranged into recognizably glandular structures. Grade 1 tumors form almost normal glands but these are progressively lost through the grades. By grade 5, tumors are characterized by sheets of undifferentiated cancer cells. In individual patients, the prognosis worsens with the progressive loss of glandular differentiation. Because prostate cancers often have a heterogeneous histological pattern, the Gleason score is calculated by the summation of the grades of the two predominant areas. Adapted from Gleason DF. The Veteran's Administration Cooperative Urologic Research Group: Histologic grading and clinical staging of prostatic carcinoma. In: Tannenbaum M, ed. *Urologic Pathology: The Prostate.* Philadelphia: Lea and Febiger, 1977:171–98.

are then summed to produce the Gleason score. More recently, the grouping of Gleason scores has been introduced, more accurately conveying the risk/aggressiveness of a cancer and allowing better counseling of patients. The system is described in more detail below.

Because prostate cancers are often heterogeneous, the numbers of the two most widely represented grades are added to produce the Gleason score (e.g. 3 + 4), which provides useful prognostic information. Occasionally, more than two grades are observed in prostatectomy or biopsy specimens, the least common being known as the tertiary grade. If the tertiary grade has a high score (4 or 5), the patient has increased risk of disease progression even if the primary and secondary grades are lower, and the tertiary rather than the secondary grade informs the score.

In 2015, a consensus conference of the International Society of Uropathology proposed a new Gleason grade grouping, which ranges from 1 to 5, 1 being the most indolent and 5 the most aggressive. Table 1.4 shows the allocation of the scores to the grade groups. The higher the Gleason grade group, the greater the likelihood that primary treatment with radical prostatectomy will fail, validating this method of reporting prostate cancer grade (Figure 1.5).

TABLE 1.4

**The Gleason grading system**

| Grade group | Gleason score | Morphological pattern |
|---|---|---|
| 1 | ≤ 6 | Only individual, discrete, well-formed glands |
| 2 | 3 + 4 = 7 | Predominantly well-formed glands, with a lesser component of poorly formed, fused or cribriform glands |
| 3 | 4 + 3 = 7 | Predominantly poorly formed, fused or cribriform glands, with a lesser component of well-formed glands* |

CONTINUED

TABLE 1.4 (CONTINUED)

**The Gleason grading system**

| Grade group | Gleason score | Morphological pattern |
|---|---|---|
| 4 | 8 | Only poorly formed, fused or cribriform glands; or |
| | | Predominantly well-formed glands with a lesser component that lacks glands[†]; or |
| | | Predominantly lacking glands, with a lesser component of well-formed glands[†] |
| 5 | 9–10 | Lacks gland formation (or with necrosis), with or without poorly formed, fused or cribriform glands* |

*For cases with >95% poorly formed, fused or cribriform glands, or lack of glands (or with necrosis) on a needle core or at radical prostatectomy, the component of <5% well-formed glands is not factored into the grade.
[†]Poorly formed, fused or cribriform glands can also be a more minor component.

Adapted from Kryvenko and Epstein. *Prostate* 2016;76:427–33.

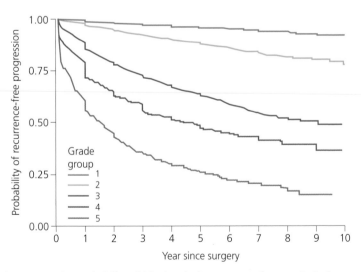

**Figure 1.5** The probability of biochemical recurrence-free survival after radical prostatectomy depends on the Gleason grade group (see Table 1.4). Adapted from Kryvenko and Epstein. *Prostate* 2016;76:427–33.

## Patterns of disease spread

Prostate cancer is also classified according to the spread of the disease, using the American Joint Committee on Cancer tumor–nodes–metastasis (TNM) system (Table 1.5). The tumor stage (T1–T4) describes the pathological development of the tumor.

- T1 represents 'incidental' status, in which the tumor is discovered after transurethral resection of the prostate (TURP) or, more commonly, by PSA testing, and is not detectable by palpation or ultrasonography.
- T2 represents a cancer that is palpable but still confined to the prostate gland.
- T3 represents a cancer that has extended through the prostate capsule into the surrounding fat or seminal vesicles.
- T4 represents advanced disease, where the tumor has invaded neighboring organs (Figure 1.6).

The nodal stages (N0–N1) and metastatic stages (M0–M1c) reflect the clinical progression of the disease. Metastases are most common in the lymph nodes (N1) and bones (M1b); the lungs and other soft tissues are less commonly involved.

It is not currently possible to distinguish unambiguously between tumors that will remain latent throughout the patient's life and those that will definitely progress to clinical disease. Studies of incidental carcinomas diagnosed after TURP suggest that the median time to progression for T1b tumors (high-volume: moderately or poorly differentiated) is 4.75 years, compared with 13.5 years for T1a tumors (low-volume; well-differentiated) (Figure 1.7). Thus, elderly men with T1a tumors are most appropriately managed by active surveillance alone (see page 60), whereas for younger men with T1b disease, options for more aggressive, potentially curative, therapy can be discussed.

TABLE 1.5

**The TNM classification of prostate cancer (2010)**

**Primary tumor**

Tx     Primary tumor cannot be assessed

T0     No evidence of primary tumor

T1     Clinically inapparent tumor not palpable or visible by imaging

      T1a   Incidental; histological finding in $\leq$ 5% of tissue resected

      T1b   Incidental; histological finding in > 5% of tissue resected

      T1c   Identified by needle biopsy (e.g. because of elevated PSA)

T2     Tumor confined within the prostate*

      T2a   Involves $\leq$ 50% of one lobe

      T2b   Involves > 50% of one lobe but not both lobes

      T2c   Involves both lobes

T3     Tumor extends through the prostatic capsule[†]

      T3a   Extracapsular extension (unilateral or bilateral)

      T3b   Invades seminal vesicle(s)

T4     Tumor is fixed or invades adjacent structures other than seminal vesicles: bladder neck, external sphincter, rectum, levator muscles and/or pelvic wall

| **Regional lymph nodes** | **Distant metastasis[‡]** |
|---|---|
| Nx   Cannot be assessed | Mx   Cannot be assessed |
| N0   No metastasis | M0   No metastasis |
| N1   Metastasis | M1   Metastasis |
| | M1a   Non-regional lymph node(s) |
| | M1b   Bone(s) |
| | M1c   Other site(s) |

*Tumor found in one or both lobes by needle biopsy, but not palpable or visible by imaging, is classified as T1c.
[†]Invasion into the prostatic apex or into (but not beyond) the prostatic capsule is not classified as T3, but as T2.
[‡]When $\geq$ 1 site of metastasis, the most advanced category should be used.
PSA, prostate-specific antigen; TNM, tumor–nodes–metastasis.

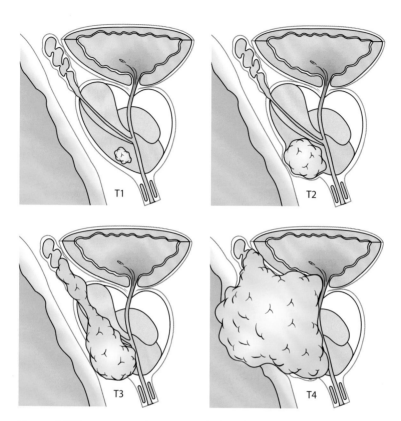

**Figure 1.6** The tumor–nodes–metastasis (TNM) system recognizes four stages of local tumor growth: T1 (incidental); T2 (confined within the prostate); T3 (extending through the prostatic capsule); T4 (invading neighboring organs).

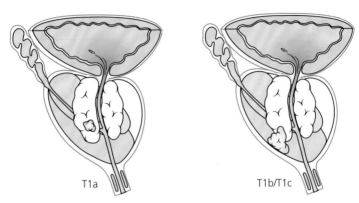

T1a          T1b/T1c

**Figure 1.7** Incidental carcinoma of the prostate is unsuspected cancer diagnosed at transurethral resection of the prostate. T1a cancers are small, well-differentiated lesions involving less than 5% of resected tissue. T1b cancers are larger, involve more than 5% of the resected chippings and are less well differentiated. T1c cancers detected by prostate-specific antigen testing are usually greater than 0.5 cm$^3$ in volume and moderately well differentiated.

---

**Key points – epidemiology and pathophysiology**

- Prostate cancer is soon likely to supersede lung cancer as the most common cause of cancer death in men in western countries, as fewer men smoke and the population is aging.
- Age is the greatest risk factor but race, family history, western-style diet and obesity also have an effect.
- Most prostate cancers are adenocarcinomas arising in the peripheral zone of the gland.
- Prostate cancers are graded according to the Gleason system, which carries prognostic significance.

## Key references

Albertsen PC, Hanley JA, Fine J. 20-year outcomes following conservative management of clinically localized prostate cancer. *JAMA* 2005;293:2095–101.

Andriole GL, Bostwick DG, Brawley OW et al. Effect of dutasteride on the risk of prostate cancer. *N Engl J Med* 2010;362:1192–202.

Bancroft EK, Page EC, Castro E et al. Targeted prostate cancer screening in *BRCA1* and *BRCA2* mutation carriers: results from the initial screening round of the IMPACT study. *Eur Urol* 2014;66:489–99 [Erratum in: *Eur Urol* 2015;67:e126].

Barocas DA, Mallin K, Graves AJ et al. Effect of the USPSTF Grade D Recommendation against Screening for Prostate Cancer on Incident Prostate Cancer Diagnoses in the United States. *J Urol* 2015;194:1587–93

Calle EE, Rodriguez C, Walker-Thurmond K, Thun MJ. Overweight, obesity, and mortality from cancer in a prospectively studied cohort of U.S. adults. *N Engl J Med* 2003;348:1625–38.

Epstein JI, Egevad L, Amin MB et al; Grading Committee. The 2014 International Society of Urological Pathology (ISUP) consensus conference on Gleason grading of prostatic carcinoma: definition of grading patterns and proposal for a new grading system. *Am J Surg Pathol* 2016;40:244–52.

Giovannucci E, Liu Y, Platz EA et al. Risk factors for prostate cancer incidence and progression in the health professionals follow-up study. *Int J Cancer* 2007;121:1571–8.

Kiciński M, Vangronsveld J, Nawrot TS. An epidemiological reappraisal of the familial aggregation of prostate cancer: a meta-analysis. *PLoS One* 2011;6:e27130.

Kryvenko ON and Epstein JI. Changes in prostate cancer grading: including a new patient-centric grading system. *Prostate* 2016;76:427–33.

Mitra AV, Bancroft EK, Barbachano Y et al. Targeted prostate cancer screening in men with mutations in *BRCA1* and *BRCA2* detects aggressive prostate cancer: preliminary analysis of the results of the IMPACT study. *BJU Int* 2011;107:28–39.

Raymond VM, Mukherjee B, Wang F et al. Elevated risk of prostate cancer among men with Lynch syndrome. *J Clin Oncol* 2013;31:1713–18.

Zheng SL, Sun J, Wiklund F et al. Cumulative association of five genetic variants with prostate cancer. *N Engl J Med* 2008;358:910–19.

### Effect on development of prostate cancer

**Diet and lifestyle** are clearly linked to the development of prostate cancer. The effects of obesity and a western-style diet as risk factors for the development of prostate cancer were mentioned in Chapter 1. A large number of studies have evaluated the effects of dietary manipulation/supplementation in reducing the incidence of prostate cancer; the current evidence is summarized in Table 2.1.

Although randomized clinical trials have provided some indication that selenium and vitamin E have a protective effect, a large chemoprevention study (the Selenium and Vitamin E Cancer Prevention Trial [SELECT]), designed to determine whether they reduced the likelihood of prostate cancer when used singly or in combination, was ended prematurely because of disappointingly negative results. Cohort studies show that lycopene (in tomatoes) and isoflavonoids (found in soy products) may be associated with a decrease in the incidence of prostate cancer. Evidence for other dietary supplements is weak.

A recently published but slightly dubious cohort study on risk factors for prostate cancer reported that having more than seven sexual partners increased the risk by 100%, and having more than five orgasms per month increased the risk by 59%. However, there is no evidence that reducing these factors reverses the risk!

**Chemoprevention** refers to the use of drugs to reduce the risk of cancer. The 5α-reductase inhibitor finasteride has been shown to reduce the incidence of prostate cancer by 24.8% compared with placebo over a 7-year period, although at the cost of a small but significant increase in sexual side effects. However, this is counterbalanced by the finding that a small proportion of cancers in the finasteride group tended to be more aggressive than those in the placebo group, although this may have been an artifact of taking biopsies from the smaller prostates in the active treatment arm

TABLE 2.1

**Effects of dietary manipulation to reduce the incidence of prostate cancer**

### Strength of evidence: Medium (single-arm study)

*Calcium* (dietary supplements, dairy products)

MSE – Reported to increase risk by up to 70% in some studies

Comment – Conflicting study results but many also show no increased risk

*Fish oils* (oily fish)

MSE – Conflicting data: recent SELECT study suggested 43% increased risk in men with highest blood levels of omega-3 fatty acids

Comment – SELECT study did not assess participants' diet or use of supplements. Other studies suggest omega-3 fatty acids from marine sources have a protective role. No clear conclusions can be drawn at present

*Lycopene* (tomatoes, watermelon, pink grapefruit, guava)

MSE – 15–20% reduction, increasing to 25% if > 2 servings of tomato product/week

Comment – Better effect with cooked or processed tomato products (e.g. tomato sauce)

*Selenium* (grains, fish, meat, poultry, dairy products)

MSE – Approximately 50% reduction with 200 µg daily in some studies; excessive intake can be toxic

Comment – Some evidence of effect, particularly in those with low PSA levels and low plasma selenium levels, but results from a large randomized controlled trial were disappointing

*Soy/isoflavonoids* (soy products)

MSE – Up to 70% reduction if > 1 serving of soy milk daily

Comment – No strong evidence but lower level evidence consistently supports an effect

*Vitamin E* (supplements)

MSE – Approximately 30% reduction with 50 mg daily

Comment – Some suggestion of an effect, but results from a large randomized controlled trial were disappointing

CONTINUED

TABLE 2.1 (CONTINUED)

**Effects of dietary manipulation to reduce the incidence of prostate cancer**

**Strength of evidence: Poor (anecdotal)**

*Saturated fat* (saturated fats, including red meat and dairy)

MSE – 10–30% increase

Comment – Associations with total fat, saturated fat, meat and linoleic acid have been reported

*Vitamin D* (supplements, sunlight)

MSE – Not established

Comment – No substantial evidence to support an effect

*Zinc* (dietary supplements)

MSE – Not established but concerns that supplements may increase risk

Comment – Epidemiological and experimental data are conflicting

MSE, maximum suggested effect.

resulting from the shrinkage effect of finasteride. A 2013 study reported that there was no difference in the overall survival (OS) rate, or survival after a diagnosis of prostate cancer, between the placebo-treated and finasteride-treated patients after 18 years of follow-up.

Another 5α-reductase inhibitor, dutasteride, has been evaluated for its effect on the occurrence of prostate cancer in the REDUCE study (Reduction by Dutasteride of Prostate Cancer Events). Dutasteride resulted in a 23% reduction in the development of prostate cancer, mainly by suppressing the well-differentiated cancers, with only a slight (statistically insignificant) increase in Gleason pattern 7 or 8–10 poorly differentiated tumors. It also effectively treated the symptoms arising from benign prostatic hyperplasia (BPH). Neither of these compounds were approved by the regulatory authorities for chemoprevention.

Statins have also been reported to have some chemopreventative properties although the evidence is weak and conflicting: a recent review found that only eight of 43 studies reported a positive association between statin use and a reduction in the development or progression of prostate cancer.

## Effect on progression

Very few trials have investigated the effect of diet and lifestyle change on prostate cancer progression. Table 2.2 outlines the current body of evidence. In addition, a large number of compounds – many of them herbal – have been tested in the laboratory and show potential; these include green tea and other polyphenols, resveratrol from red wine, vitamin D, epilobium and *Serenoa repens* (saw palmetto).

TABLE 2.2

**Effect of diet and lifestyle on prostate cancer progression**

| Factor and effect | Comment |
| --- | --- |
| **Exercise** | |
| No clear evidence but suspected to be of benefit | Performance index is an independent prognostic indicator in clinical trials |
| **Low-fat diet** | |
| Possible reduction in cancer growth | Low level of clinical benefit based on animal and human biomarker studies |
| **Fish oils/omega-3 fatty acids** | |
| Possible reduction in cancer growth | Based on a cohort study and an animal study |
| **Lycopene** | |
| Reasonable evidence of a reduction in PSA and tumor size | Two servings per week associated with 20% risk reduction from cohort and animal studies |
| **Pomegranate juice** | |
| Possible reduction in PSA rise after prostate cancer recurrence | Based on low-level evidence from phase II trials |
| **Soy/isoflavonoids** | |
| Inconclusive evidence of any benefit | In-vitro results favorable but an animal study was not supportive |

PSA, prostate-specific antigen.

It must be remembered that cardiovascular disease is still the primary cause of death in men, with or without prostate cancer, and heart-healthy lifestyle choices will reduce mortality in men with prostate cancer. These include improving lipid profiles, decreasing obesity and increasing physical fitness. A healthy diet and regular vigorous exercise may help protect the individual against various forms of cancer, in addition to decreasing the risk of death from cardiovascular causes.

Evidence for a beneficial effect of exercise on prostate cancer-specific mortality is also increasing, and post-diagnosis recreational activity has been shown to significantly lower prostate cancer-specific mortality. The mechanism many not be merely related to decreased sedentary activity, however, as there was no association between sedentary activity and increased mortality.

---

**Key points – diet, lifestyle and chemoprevention**

- In one trial, the 5α-reductase inhibitor, dutasteride, reduced the incidence of prostate cancer by about one-quarter over 4 years and also relieved symptoms of benign prostatic hyperplasia (BPH), but slightly increased the incidence of high-grade cancer. Finasteride produced similar results.
- Men should be advised/supported to lower lipid profiles, address obesity and increase exercise and fitness as part of a strategy to cut the risk of cardiovascular disease and associated death, and, possibly, prostate cancer.

## Key references

Andriole GL, Bostwick DG, Brawley OW et al. Effect of dutasteride on the risk of prostate cancer. *N Engl J Med* 2010;362:1192–202.

Babcook MA, Joshi A, Montellano JA et al. Statin use in prostate cancer: an update. *Nutr Metab Insights* 2016;14;43–50.

Cohen YC, Liu KS, Heyden NL et al. Detection bias due to the effect of finasteride on prostate volume: a modeling approach for analysis of the Prostate Cancer Prevention Trial. *J Natl Cancer Inst* 2007;99:1366–74.

Giovannucci E, Liu Y, Platz EA et al. Risk factors for prostate cancer incidence and progression in the health professionals follow-up study. *Int J Cancer* 2007;121:1571–8.

Lippmani SM, Klein EA, Goodman PJ et al. Effect of selenium and vitamin E on risk of prostate cancer and other cancers: the Selenium and Vitamin E Cancer Prevention Trial (SELECT). *JAMA* 2009;301:39–51.

Lucia MS, Epstein JI, Goodman PJ et al. Finasteride and high-grade prostate cancer in the Prostate Cancer Prevention Trial. *J Natl Cancer Inst* 2007;99:1375–83.

Miller EC, Giovannucci E, Erdman JW Jr et al. Tomato products, lycopene, and prostate cancer risk. *Urol Clin North Am* 2002;29:83–93.

Nair-Shalliker V, Yap S, Nunez C et al. Adult body size, sexual history and adolescent sexual development may predict risk of developing prostate cancer: Results from the New South Wales Cancer Lifestyle and Evaluation of Risk Study (CLEAR). *Int J Cancer* 2017;140:565–74.

Thompson IM, Goodman PJ, Tangen CM et al. The influence of finasteride on the development of prostate cancer. *N Engl J Med* 2003;349:215–24.

Thompson IM, Goodman PJ, Tangen CM et al. Long-term survival in the Prostate Cancer Prevention Trial. *N Engl J Med* 2013;369:603–10.

Virtamo J, Pietinen P, Huttunen JK et al. Incidence of cancer and mortality following α-tocopherol and β-carotene supplementation: a postintervention follow-up. *JAMA* 2003;290:476–85.

The past decade has seen a significant downward shift in the stage at presentation of prostate cancer in most countries. Historically, most men with clinically significant disease presented with a combination of weight loss, bone pain, lethargy and bladder outflow obstruction, attributable to locally advanced or metastatic disease. More commonly today, early disease is detected incidentally from measurement of prostate-specific antigen (PSA) in younger, asymptomatic men; occasionally it is an incidental histological finding following transurethral resection of the prostate (TURP) for benign obstructive symptoms. This earlier presentation has posed dilemmas concerning management, and the increasing life expectancy of patients (Figure 3.1) underscores the urgent need for effective evidence-based diagnosis and treatment regimens.

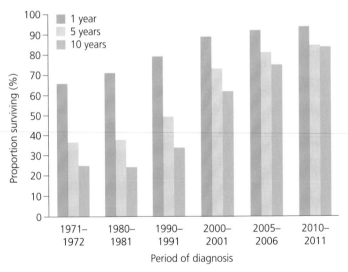

**Figure 3.1** Relative survival (%) at 1, 5 and 10 years after diagnosis of prostate cancer in England and Wales (men diagnosed in six periods from 1971 to 2011). Reproduced from Cancer Research UK. www.cancerresearchuk.org/cancer-info/cancerstats/survival/common-cancers, last accessed 07 March 2017.

## Early detection

In general, the earlier prostate cancer is detected, the better the outlook in terms of cure or arresting cancer progression. However, we always need to be cognizant of the risk of over-diagnosis and potential over-treatment. Most patients in whom prostate cancer is suspected are identified on the basis of abnormal findings on digital rectal exam (DRE) or, more commonly, by raised levels of PSA. An increasing majority of patients present simply with an isolated increase in PSA.

**Digital rectal exam** is the simplest, safest and most cost-effective means of detecting prostate cancer, provided that the tumor is posteriorly situated and is sufficiently large to be palpable. The test can be performed with the patient either in the left lateral position or standing and leaning forwards; with either approach only the posterior portion of the gland is palpable (Figure 3.2). In addition to providing information on the size of the prostate, DRE can reveal a number of features that may indicate prostate cancer (Table 3.1), although only approximately one-third of suspicious prostatic nodules are confirmed as malignant when analyzed histologically after prostate biopsy (Table 3.2).

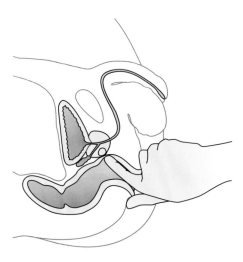

**Figure 3.2** Digital rectal exam is an essential clinical test in the detection and diagnosis of prostate cancer.

TABLE 3.1

**Digital rectal exam findings that may indicate prostate cancer**

- A nodule within one or both lobes of the gland
- Induration of part or all of the prostate
- Asymmetry of the gland
- Lack of mobility due to adhesion to surrounding tissue
- Palpable seminal vesicles

TABLE 3.2

**Other causes of digital rectal exam abnormalities**

- Benign prostatic hyperplasia
- Prostatic calculi
- Prostatitis (particularly granulomatous prostatitis)
- Ejaculatory duct abnormalities
- Seminal vesicle abnormalities
- Rectal mucosal polyp or tumor

**Prostate-specific antigen** is a glycoprotein responsible for liquefying semen. Tissue barriers become compromised in prostatic disease, including cancer, allowing more PSA to enter the bloodstream (Figure 3.3). Measurement of serum PSA is still the most effective single screening test for early detection of prostate cancer; in fact, it can detect more than twice as many prostate cancers as DRE, and the predictive value is increased further if the measurement is combined (as it always should be) with DRE. PSA determination is also useful in staging prostate cancer and has particular value in evaluating the response to therapy and in alerting clinicians to the possibility of recurrence (see Chapter 4).

Approximately 25% of men with PSA levels above 4 ng/mL harbor some form of prostate cancer, and the risk increases to more than 60% in men with PSA levels above 10 ng/mL. Causes of PSA elevation in the absence of prostate cancer are given in Table 3.3. A study of

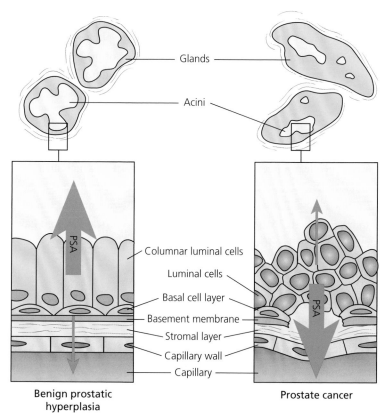

Glands

Acini

Columnar luminal cells

Luminal cells

Basal cell layer

Basement membrane

Stromal layer

Capillary wall

Capillary

PSA

PSA

Benign prostatic
hyperplasia

Prostate cancer

**Figure 3.3** Normally, there are significant tissue barriers between the lumen of the prostate gland and the capillary bed. These barriers are compromised in prostatic disease, particularly cancer, and serum PSA levels rise.

TABLE 3.3

**Causes of PSA elevation**

- Prostate cancer
- Perineal or prostatic trauma
- Benign prostatic hyperplasia
- Recent ejaculation
- Prostatitis
- Cycling
- Urinary tract infection

prostate cancer prevention, in which all men in the placebo group underwent biopsy, reported a significant incidence of prostate cancer in men with PSA levels between 0.5 and 4 ng/mL and normal DRE (Table 3.4). The median PSA and 95th percentile values for the 'normal' population at each age group are presented in Table 3.5. As shown by the data in Table 3.4, a significant percentage of men with PSA values below the 95th percentile will harbor prostate cancer. There is no clear agreement on the best PSA cut-off at which men should undergo biopsy: a cut-off of 4.0 ng/mL has been used in the past, but a cut-off at 2.5 ng/mL would double the cancer detection rate from 18% to 36% in men younger than 60 years and would have a minimal negative effect on specificity.

TABLE 3.4

**Likelihood of prostate cancer on biopsy in men with normal digital rectal exam**

| PSA level (ng/mL) | Risk of prostate cancer on biopsy (%) |
|---|---|
| < 0.5 | 6.6 |
| 0.5–1.0 | 10.1 |
| 1.1–2.0 | 17.0 |
| 2.1–3.0 | 23.9 |
| 3.1–4.0 | 26.9 |

PSA, prostate-specific antigen. Data from Thompson et al., 2004.

TABLE 3.5

**Age-related PSA levels in a male population**

| Age range (years) | Median PSA (ng/mL) | 95th percentile |
|---|---|---|
| 40–49 | 0.7 | 2.5 |
| 50–59 | 0.9 | 3.5 |
| 60–69 | 1.3 | 4.5 |
| 70–79 | 1.8 | 6.5 |

PSA, prostate-specific antigen. Data from Oesterling JE et al. *JAMA* 1993;270:860–4.

Many men with mildly elevated PSA levels have benign prostatic hyperplasia (BPH) rather than prostate cancer, however, so it is clear that PSA is not a perfect test. Several concepts have been developed to improve the clinical value of the test in the detection of early prostate cancer. These 'PSA derivatives' include PSA density, PSA velocity, age-specific reference ranges and differential assay of the different molecular forms of serum PSA. All of these have been proposed in attempts to improve the utility of PSA in the detection of early prostate cancer at a curable stage and to reduce the number of negative transrectal biopsies.

*PSA density* is calculated by dividing the total PSA by the prostate volume (usually measured by transrectal ultrasonography). A PSA density above 0.15 ng/mL has been shown to increase the specificity of the PSA test. This modification does, however, have many potential sources of error, such as in the volume calculation, assay variability and sampling bias (Figure 3.4).

*PSA velocity* refers to the rate of PSA change, usually over 1 or 2 years, based on a minimum of three readings. A velocity above 0.75 ng/mL/year has been used to predict the presence of prostate cancer. However, recent studies have shown that the average PSA velocity in men without prostate cancer is 0.03 ng/mL/year, compared

PSA 8.0 ng/mL
Volume 40 cm³

PSA 8.0 ng/mL
Volume 80 cm³

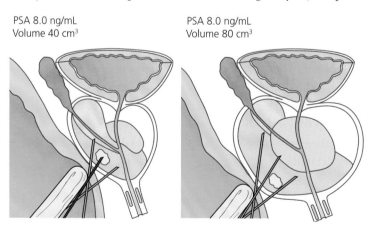

**Figure 3.4** Biopsies taken from a larger prostate with a lower PSA density are less likely to sample the cancer than those taken from a smaller prostate with a higher PSA density.

with 0.4 ng/mL/year in men ultimately diagnosed with prostate cancer. A PSA velocity of 0.35–0.4 ng/mL/year is largely recommended as the threshold at which biopsy is recommended, even if the actual PSA level is within the normal range. Problems associated with PSA velocity include inaccuracy of velocity calculation over short time periods, and too few measurements being made (PSA levels show natural fluctuation, such as after ejaculation).

*Age-specific reference ranges* are predicated on the increase in serum PSA level with age. As a result, the reference range is corrected for the patient's age (see Table 3.5). This practice increases positive-predictive values from 37% to 42% but decreases cancer detection when compared with a cut-off of 4.0 ng/mL. Studies have shown that age-specific median PSA values may be more useful than age-specific cut-offs, as young men with a PSA above their age-specific median value but below a biopsy threshold of 2.5 ng/mL have an 8–14-fold increased risk of developing prostate cancer. Figure 3.5 shows the problem with using an age-specific cut-off rather than a standard cut-off for all ages – too many cancers are missed in older men (in whom prevalence is considerably higher).

*Molecular forms.* PSA exists in the serum in several molecular forms; most of it is bound to protein but some is unbound or 'free'. Studies show that patients with BPH but not prostate cancer have a higher amount of free PSA, whereas men with prostate cancer appear to have a greater amount of PSA complexed with $\alpha_1$-antichymotrypsin. Measuring the concentration of these different molecular forms in the serum is a clinically useful way to distinguish between BPH and early prostate cancer. The currently accepted cut-off for free:total PSA is 0.15. Men with ratios below this should be considered for further investigation, including MRI and/or transrectal or transperineal prostatic biopsy.

**Prostate Health Index.** This index, which was approved in the USA in 2013, is a mathematical formula that combines total PSA, free PSA and [–2]proPSA (an isoform of PSA produced primarily in the peripheral zone of the prostate). This test has performed better than conventional PSA and free PSA for predicting overall and high-grade

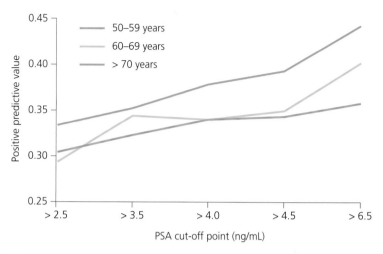

**Figure 3.5** At any given PSA cut-off, the positive predictive value is higher for older men than for younger men, because of the increased prevalence of prostate cancer with age. Although raising the PSA cut-off will increase the positive predictive value further for older men, a proportion of men will have false-negative tests and the overall detection rate will be reduced.

cancer in a number of studies. However, it does not add any predictive value if MRI is also used.

*PCA3* (**Prostate CAncer gene 3**) is a piece of non-coding RNA that is only present in the prostate. It has value as a potential biomarker because levels in prostate cancer tissue are greatly increased (up to 66-fold) but are not increased in benign conditions such as BPH. The *PCA3* test also appears to be reasonably sensitive, detecting increases in tissue samples containing fewer than 10% cancer cells. *PCA3* score is positively associated with the probability of a positive biopsy, and the relationship appears to be unaffected by prostate volume, prostatitis, number of prior biopsies or 5α-reductase inhibitor treatment for BPH. *PCA3* is becoming incorporated into diagnostic nomograms, and research into its role in prostate cancer prediction and monitoring is continuing, although it is not yet widely used in clinical practice. The value of the *PCA3* test is likely to be in reducing the number of repeat biopsies. The use of *PCA3* in this setting has a negative predictive value of 90% and has been shown to help reduce the number of biopsies performed in men who have persistently elevated PSA after a first biopsy. The value has also been shown to correlate with the Gleason score of the diagnosed cancer.

## Screening

The value of PSA screening in men who are asymptomatic for prostate cancer is still highly controversial (Table 3.6). As described in Chapter 1, there is a great discrepancy between the incidence of clinically significant disease and the prevalence of microscopic disease, and the identification of men in whom disease progression is probable remains inexact. The current evidence to support PSA screening is as follows.

- Non-randomized data show that, since the advent of PSA screening in the USA and Europe, the proportion of men presenting with advanced prostate cancer has decreased, as has prostate cancer mortality.

TABLE 3.6

**Screening for prostate cancer**

Advantages

- Simple tests available (PSA and DRE)
- Detects early, potentially curable, lesions
- Reassures those who are screened as negative
- Reduces mortality by up to 56%

Disadvantages

- False-positive findings cause anxiety
- Biopsy guided by transrectal ultrasonography carries a 2% risk of serious infective complications and causes anxiety
- Expensive
- Some small slow-growing tumors may be treated unnecessarily, and treatment has side effects

DRE, digital rectal exam; PSA, prostate-specific antigen.

- In one randomized study, men with clinically significant prostate cancer treated with radical prostatectomy had a 56% reduction in the risk of premature death from prostate cancer compared with conservative management.
- The PSA test and DRE are simple to perform, and prostate biopsy has a relatively low complication rate (2–4%).
  Disadvantages to screening include the following.
- Clinically insignificant cancers that may be better left undetected may be diagnosed and treated.
- The PIVOT trial showed little benefit of surgery compared with watchful waiting in men with lower-risk cancers.
- A large proportion of men who have a biopsy do not harbor prostate cancer, and biopsies have associated morbidity because of the risk of post-biopsy infection.
- The screening process may generate anxiety.
- The treatment of prostate cancer is associated with significant morbidity.

The 2013 American Urological Association (AUA) guidelines recommend against PSA screening in men under 40 years of age, and do not recommend routine screening in men aged 40–54 years who are considered to be at average risk, as men of this age were not included in the randomized screening studies. Decisions about screening should be individualized for men younger than 55 years who have risk factors for prostate cancer (see page 8). The strongest evidence for a benefit of screening is in men aged 55–69 years; the AUA guidelines recommend that decisions about screening for men aged 55–69 should be shared between the fully informed man and his clinician, and based on the individual's values and preferences.

Early results from two large randomized studies and longer-term results from a third randomized study have been reported. The larger European study (the European Randomized Study of Screening for Prostate Cancer [ERSPC]) randomized men to screening at 4-yearly intervals or no screening. A biopsy was mandated if the PSA was above 3.0 ng/mL or DRE was abnormal. This study reported a 27% reduction in prostate cancer mortality at a median follow-up of 9 years. Unfortunately, however, the number needed to treat to save one death (NNT) was as high as 48. A report on a subset of men in this trial from Gothenburg, Sweden, with a median 14-year follow-up, showed a higher cumulative incidence of prostate cancer among the screened population (Figure 3.6). Prostate cancer mortality was reduced by 44% in those randomized to screening. In men who actually attended screening, prostate cancer mortality was reduced by 56%. With longer follow-up, the NNT was reduced to 12.

In contrast, the smaller US study (the Prostate, Lung, Colorectal, and Ovarian [PLCO] Cancer Screening Trial) did not find a mortality benefit at a shorter follow-up, although this trial was flawed because the control arm received almost as much PSA screening as the screening arm.

A recently updated Cochrane meta-analysis of five randomized controlled trials concluded that screening did not result in a statistically significant reduction in prostate cancer-specific mortality when all populations of all studies were included (risk ratio 1.0 [0.86–1.17]) (Figure 3.7). In 2012, the US Preventive Services Task Force (USPSTF) published its recommendation advising against PSA screening in all men (following a draft recommendation in 2011).

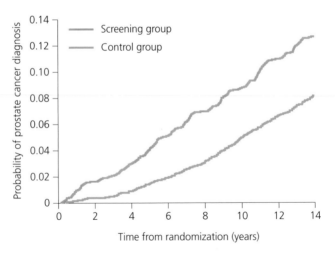

**Figure 3.6** Cumulative incidence of prostate cancer in men randomized to screening or observation in the Gothenburg Randomised Population-based Prostate-cancer Screening Trial. Reproduced with permission from Hugosson et al. *Lancet Oncol* 2010;11:725–32.

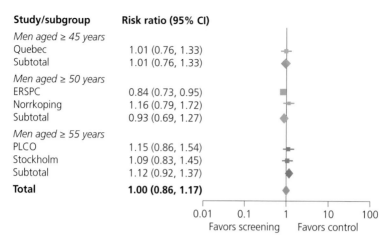

**Figure 3.7** Forest plot showing the risk ratios for prostate-cancer mortality in men screened for the disease versus controls: a meta-analysis of five randomized trials. ERSPC, European Randomized Study of Screening for Prostate Cancer; PLCO, Protate, Lung, Colorectal and Ovarian cancer screening trial. Adapted from Ilic et al. 2013.

Since then there have been a number of reports of decreased prostate biopsies, fewer diagnoses of low-risk prostate cancer and fewer radical prostatectomies in the USA. However, there have also been reports that the cancer volume on biopsy and grade of cancers are increasing. It is yet to be confirmed whether or not men are now presenting with later stages than before the USPSTF recommendation.

Measurement of PSA in early midlife (40–55 years) can identify a small group of men at risk of prostate cancer metastasis several decades later: men who have a PSA in the highest 10th percentile for their age group have a 3–10-fold higher risk of metastasis 15 years later. Men with a PSA above 1.0 ng/mL in this age group have also been found to be at higher risk of developing metastatic prostate cancer and it has been suggested that they should be invited for regular PSA tests.

In the future, it seems likely that screening will be focused on men who are genetically most susceptible to prostate cancer. More than 100 'prostate cancer susceptibility genes' have been discovered. Men who are at risk because of mutations in these genes could be targeted for screening.

Right now, the family physician has an important role in assessing the likely benefits and risks for individual patients according to their age and life expectancy; appropriate counseling of the patient and his immediate family is an essential element of this process.

The decision to perform a biopsy in any man with an abnormal PSA or DRE should not be based simply on a single PSA value but on a patient's risk factors, including race, family history, previous PSA values, previous biopsy results and assessment of comorbidities and life expectancy. The patient's own informed preferences should be central in the decision-making process.

## Clinical symptoms

Patients with prostate cancer may present with a variety of symptoms (Table 3.7), many of which overlap with those of BPH.

Localized cancer is generally asymptomatic. Men most often present with symptoms of BPH that are unrelated to the cancer. These

TABLE 3.7

**Clinical presentation/symptoms of local and locally invasive prostate cancer**

| Local disease | Locally invasive disease |
|---|---|
| • Asymptomatic | • Hematuria |
| • Elevated PSA | • Dysuria |
| • Symptoms of benign prostatic hypertrophy: | • Perineal and suprapubic pain |
|   – Weak stream | • Erectile dysfunction |
|   – Hesitancy | • Incontinence |
|   – Sensation of incomplete emptying | • Loin pain or anuria resulting from obstruction of the ureters |
|   – Frequency | • Symptoms of renal failure |
|   – Urgency | • Hemospermia |
|   – Urge incontinence | • Rectal symptoms, including tenesmus |
|   – Urinary tract infection | |

symptoms occur when benign prostatic tissue compresses and obstructs the urethra, resulting in frequency, hesitancy and poor urine flow. Prostate cancer may also present as an 'incidental' finding after TURP (Figure 3.8); nowadays, fewer than 10% of men undergoing TURP for BPH are found to have microscopic foci of prostate cancer.

**Locally advanced cancers** (usually palpable by DRE) may cause symptoms resulting from local extension of the tumor, such as irritative symptoms (frequency, urgency) due to invasion of the

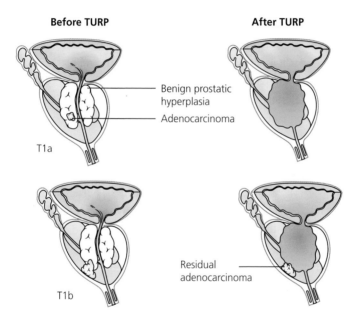

**Figure 3.8** Prostate cancer is found in resected chips of prostate tissue obtained during transurethral resection of the prostate (TURP) in up to 10% of cases. About two-thirds of the cancers are well-differentiated T1a lesions involving fewer than 5% of the chips. The remaining lesions are T1b cancers that have larger volume and are less well differentiated. A number of potential sampling errors are inherent in the diagnosis of prostate cancer at TURP. T1a tumors that are confined to the transition zone may be completely excised, whereas significant amounts of T1b tumors may remain after the procedure.

bladder trigone and pelvic nerves. Involvement of the perineal or suprapubic nerves can lead to pain. The possibility of prostate cancer should therefore be considered in the investigation of prostatitis-like symptoms.

Hematuria can occur as a result of local spread of the cancer into the urethra or bladder, and loin pain can be caused by ureteric obstruction and hydronephrosis. Symptoms of bladder outlet obstruction can occur when a large tumor obstructs the bladder outlet, similar to BPH. Invasion of the urethral sphincter or, much more commonly, surgery itself may cause urinary incontinence. It is important to exclude the possibility that incontinence is a result of chronic urinary retention with overflow, which may be treatable with procedures such as TURP. Constipation, tenesmus and rectal bleeding occur if the enlarged prostate distorts the rectum. Invasion of the seminal vesicles may occasionally result in hemospermia but this is not a common presenting symptom. In rare cases, prostate cancer may extend into the corpora cavernosa.

**Metastatic disease.** The most common presenting symptoms are shown in Table 3.8. Pain resulting from bony metastases, particularly in the pelvis and lumbar spine, is the major symptom; thus, the sudden onset of progressive low back or pelvic pain is an important diagnostic feature of metastatic prostate cancer. Pathological fractures may also occur, particularly affecting the neck of the femur. Metastases within the vertebrae, sometimes leading to spinal cord compression, are not uncommon and may produce backache or neurological symptoms in up to 12% of affected men.

Metastasis into the lymph nodes may cause their enlargement. Intra-abdominal lymph node metastasis usually begins in the obturator and internal iliac nodes, spreads to the common iliac nodes and beyond and may, with local tumors, obstruct the ureters. In advanced disease, lymphatic involvement may extend to the thoracic, cervical, inguinal and axillary nodes. Lymph node metastases may produce a number of symptoms, including palpable swellings, loin pain or anuria due to obstruction of the ureters, and swelling of the legs due to lymphedema.

TABLE 3.8

**Presenting symptoms of metastatic prostate cancer**

**Distant metastases**

- Bone pain or sciatica
- Paraplegia secondary to spinal cord compression
- Lymph node enlargement
- Loin pain or anuria due to obstruction of ureters by lymph nodes

**Widespread metastases**

- Lethargy (from anemia or uremia, for example)
- Weight loss and cachexia
- Cutaneous and bowel hemorrhage (unusual)

Systemic metastases in the liver, lungs or elsewhere may produce non-specific symptoms, such as lethargy resulting from anemia or uremia, weight loss and cachexia.

---

**Key points – screening and early detection**

- Increasingly, prostate cancer is being diagnosed on the basis of a raised prostate-specific antigen (PSA) level and subsequent investigation.
- PSA-based screening of asymptomatic men is controversial.
- A baseline PSA at age 40–55 years may assess a man's future risk of developing prostate cancer.
- More advanced disease can present with symptoms of bladder outflow obstruction, hematuria or ureteric obstruction.
- Bone metastases may cause bone pain or pathological fracture.

## Key references

Carter HB, Albertsen PC, Barry MJ et al. Early detection of prostate cancer: AUA Guideline. *J Urol* 2013;190:419–26.

Hugosson J, Carlsson S, Aus G et al. Mortality results from the Göteborg randomised population-based prostate-cancer screening trial. *Lancet Oncol* 2010;11:725–32.

Ilic D, Neuberger MM, Djulbegovic M, Dahm P. Screening for prostate cancer. *Cochrane Database Syst Rev* 2013(1):CD004720.

Schröder FH, Hugosson J, Roobol MJ et al; ERSPC Investigators. Screening and prostate cancer mortality: results of the European Randomised Study of Screening for Prostate Cancer (ERSPC) at 13 years of follow-up. *Lancet* 2014;384:2027–35.

Thompson IM, Pauler DK, Goodman PJ et al. Prevalence of prostate cancer among men with a prostate-specific antigen level < or = 4.0 ng per milliliter. *N Engl J Med* 2004;350:2239–46.

US Preventive Services Task Force. *Recommendation Statement: Screening for Prostate Cancer.* www.uspreventiveservicestaskforce. org/prostatecancerscreening/ prostatefinalrs.htm, last accessed 07 March 2017.

Vickers AJ, Ulmert D, Sjoberg DD et al. Strategy for detection of prostate cancer based on relation between prostate specific antigen at age 40–55 and long term risk of metastasis: case-control study. *BMJ* 2013;346:f2023.

Once a man has undergone a prostate-specific antigen (PSA) test and digital rectal exam (DRE), a reasonable level of suspicion for the presence of prostate cancer may arise. The next step is to make the definitive diagnosis. This requires a prostate biopsy which will give definitive histological evidence of prostate cancer and also the cancer grade (Gleason grade group; see pages 14–16). Multiparametric MRI is increasingly used before biopsy to identify suspicious lesions within the prostate that would allow targeted biopsy, and may also mean that biopsy can be avoided in some men with normal MRI findings and lower levels of suspicion.

## Multiparametric MRI

Multiparametric (mp) MRI – which is based on four MRI techniques – is increasingly used to identify 'areas of interest', so that biopsies can be better targeted, and to stage prostate cancer.

**T2-weighted imaging** provides excellent zonal anatomy, and prostate cancer can be identified as a low-intensity signal (Figure 4.1), although it is more difficult to identify on T2-weighted images of the transition zone.

**Dynamic contrast-enhanced MRI** involves imaging the prostate during rapid infusion of gadolinium contrast. Prostate cancer is detected based on early enhancement and early wash-out (resulting from the greater vascularity due to increased angiogenesis). While this enhancement is typical, it is not specific; it has a sensitivity of 46–96% and specificity of 74–96% for defining prostate cancer.

**Diffusion-weighted MRI** generates maps showing the diffusion of water within tissues; water diffuses more easily in normal prostate tissue, where glands are loosely packed, than in tumor tissue, where glands are tightly

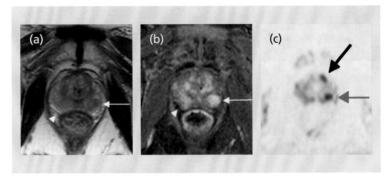

**Figure 4.1** MRI scans of a prostate gland: (a) shows suspicious areas in the left (arrow) and right (arrow head) peripheral zone on T2-weighted imaging; (b) dynamic contrast enhancement shows early contrast enhancement of the left peripheral zone lesion (arrow); (c) a diffusion-weighted image highlights the left peripheral zone lesion (red arrow) as well as a left anterior lesion (black arrow). Reproduced with permission from Iwazawa J et al. *Diagn Interv Radiol* 2011;17:243–8.

packed. This modality can also give an indication of the aggressiveness of the cancer, as highly aggressive tumors show poorer diffusion of water. Sensitivities and specificities for the detection of prostate cancer are reported to be 57–93.3% and 57–100%, respectively.

**Magnetic resonance spectroscopy** (i.e. evaluating chemical metabolites in a small volume of interest) can also improve the accuracy of staging but is not often used in clinical practice.

**Accuracy.** The combination of MRI methods is claimed to significantly improve the detection and local staging of prostate cancer by MRI, and is now widely used before prostate biopsy to target suspicious areas, and to follow up patients managed by active surveillance. Indeed, some are now arguing that prior MRI is a prerequisite to improve the accuracy of biopsy and to avoid false-negative findings. Furthermore, in cases where a biopsy is warranted, a negative finding on MRI can provide reassurance to the patient, i.e. that they don't have prostate cancer. The recently completed PROMIS study evaluated the diagnostic accuracy of an mpMRI scan followed by both template prostate mapping (TPM) biopsy and standard transrectal ultrasonography (TRUS)-guided biopsy in 576 men with suspected prostate cancer. Fewer than half (40%) of those who underwent TPM were diagnosed with aggressive cancer, and mpMRI identified 93% of the clinically significant cancers, whereas the TRUS biopsy only correctly identified 48%. Furthermore, nine out of 10 men (89%) who had a negative mpMRI scan did not have a cancer, or had a harmless cancer. The authors concluded that prior MRI avoids unnecessary TRUS biopsy in 27% of men whilst reducing the number of men who are 'over diagnosed' by 5%. If subsequent TRUS biopsy is directed by mpMRI findings, up to 18% more cases of clinically significant cancer might be detected compared with using TRUS biopsy in all patients.

## Prostate biopsy

The advent of mpMRI has changed significantly the way in which prostate biopsies are performed.

- If the MRI is normal (or is not performed), biopsies of the prostate may be performed systematically, either transrectally or transperineally.
- In men with suspicious lesions on MRI, targeted biopsies can be performed by cognitive, MRI–ultrasonography fusion or, rarely, in-bore MRI-guided biopsy (see pages 48–9).

**Transrectal ultrasonography-guided biopsy** (Figure 4.2) has been the standard method for performing prostate biopsy for decades and it is now routinely performed on an outpatient basis, after infiltration with local anesthesia. Usually 12–18 TRUS-guided biopsies are taken from different regions of the prostate using an 18-gauge needle. Antibiotics are obligatory before and after the procedure to reduce the risk of infection, currently estimated at 2–5%, although this may be rising because of increases in the antibiotic resistance of bacteria, particularly *Escherichia coli*. A quinolone is the usual choice, sometimes in combination with gentamicin or amikacin, depending on prostate size, personal preference and previous biopsy results. Patients should be warned about the risk of post-biopsy sepsis and the need for treatment if it occurs.

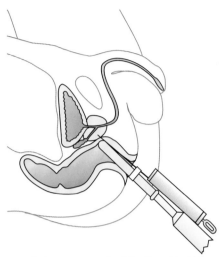

**Figure 4.2** Transrectal ultrasonography (TRUS)-guided biopsy.
An ultrasound probe is introduced into the rectum to lie adjacent to
the prostate; multiple prostatic biopsies can be taken using an automatic
biopsy gun.

**Transperineal template biopsy** (Figure 4.3) avoids the risk of sepsis
associated with the transrectal approach, and allows better sampling
of the anterior zone of the prostate, which may be under-sampled by
TRUS biopsy, particularly in large prostate glands. This transperineal
technique allows extended sampling of the gland, but requires general
anesthesia and is associated with a small but significant risk of urinary
retention.

**Cognitive targeted biopsy.** If a suspicious lesion is identified on MRI,
targeted biopsies are required to sample the area. The most simple,
but potentially least accurate, method is cognitive registration, where
the MRI is reviewed before the biopsy in order to cognitively target
the region of interest on the ultrasound image. This technique does not
require special equipment or training, but small lesions may be missed.

**MRI–ultrasound fusion targeted biopsy** uses software to overlay an
MRI scan with the suspicious lesion highlighted onto the real-time
ultrasound image during the biopsy, allowing the urologist to target

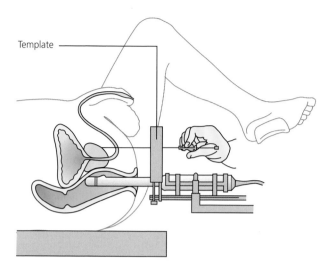

**Figure 4.3** Transperineal template biopsy is an alternative to transrectal ultrasonography that allows better sampling of the anterior prostate.

the suspicious lesion directly. However, a prospective trial found that this technique did not provide any substantial improvement in accuracy over cognitive biopsy.

**In-bore MRI-guided biopsy** involves placing the patient in the MRI gantry and performing the biopsy under real-time MRI guidance. While this is the most accurate method of targeting a suspicious lesion on MRI, the technique is cumbersome and is not clinically practicable for most patients.

**Ultrasound-guided biopsy.** Cancer within the prostate gland is not reliably apparent with ultrasonography but can occasionally present with a number of ultrasonographic abnormalities, such as abnormal echo patterns (usually hypoechoic), loss of differentiation between central and peripheral zones, asymmetry of size or shape, and capsular distortion.

Some prostate tumors are hypoechoic, but hypoechoic images may result from other causes, so the specificity of this finding for prostate cancer is only 20–25%. Assessment of local staging by TRUS imaging alone is poor. When extracapsular or seminal vesicle extension is suspected on imaging, a biopsy of the suspicious area is required for confirmation.

## Staging of localized disease

Accurate grading and staging of prostate cancer, particularly distinguishing between Gleason grades and between localized and more extensive disease, is critical for selection of the optimum treatment. Although developments in imaging techniques, especially MRI, have led to more accurate staging than can be achieved with DRE or PSA testing alone, both under- and overstaging are still common clinical problems. Thus, a need remains not only for improved staging techniques, but also for better prognostic markers that can provide an accurate indication of how the disease may behave if left untreated.

Staging of localized disease relies on the following techniques:
- DRE
- PSA measurement
- CT scanning
- mpMRI
- radionuclide bone scan
- PET/CT (with PSMA [prostate-specific prostate antigen] ligand or choline).

**Digital rectal exam** has an accuracy for staging prostate cancer of only 30–50%. Underestimation is common because small and anterior tumors are generally impalpable; false-positive findings may occur in patients with conditions such as BPH, prostatic calculi or prostatitis.

**Prostate-specific antigen determination.** A reasonable correlation between PSA levels and clinical stage (and, to a lesser extent, pathological stage) of prostate cancer is seen within overall groups of patients. However, the correlation is poorer in individual patients because of the considerable overlap between the PSA ranges associated with different stages. PSA levels above 20 ng/mL often indicate tumor extension beyond the prostatic capsule, while levels above 40 ng/mL suggest a high likelihood of bony and/or soft tissue metastases (see the Memorial Sloan-Kettering Cancer Center's pretreatment nomogram at http://nomograms.mskcc.org/Prostate/PreTreatment.aspx).

Although the serum PSA level alone may not be a precise indicator of stage on an individual basis, it can sometimes be used to eliminate some staging investigations. Men who present with newly diagnosed, well- or moderately well-differentiated prostate cancer, no skeletal symptoms and a serum PSA value of 10 ng/mL or less may not need a staging radionuclide bone scan because the probability of skeletal metastases approaches zero. However, many clinicians still like to use this test as a baseline investigation, because it may identify 'hot spots' due to conditions such as degenerative osteoarthritis that may cause confusion later, if the PSA level starts to rise. A negative scan also serves to reassure a patient that his skeleton is not involved.

**Multiparametric MRI** can be used to stage as well as detect prostate cancer. Identification of extracapsular extension or invasion into the seminal vesicles depends on the identification of regions of low signal intensity in the normally bright periprostatic fat and seminal vesicles. It may, however, depend on more subtle changes, such as asymmetry of the neurovascular bundles, irregular gland margins or capsular obliteration. The sensitivity of MRI for the detection of extracapsular extension is reported to range from 13% to 95%; accuracy is certainly higher in units with considerable experience in the interpretation of prostate images. MRI provides little advantage over CT in the evaluation of nodal metastases. However, promising results have been reported with the use of ultra-small superparamagnetic iron oxide particles as an aid to the evaluation of nodal metastases by MRI.

**Staging of metastatic disease** involves assessing the extent of bone and soft tissue involvement. The principal techniques are chest radiography, radionuclide bone scanning, CT and MRI and, more recently, [11]C-choline PET/CT and [68]Ga-PSMA PET.

*CT* of the abdomen and pelvis may be used to inform treatment decisions that depend on the presence and degree of lymph node or other soft tissue involvement. Small-volume and microscopic metastases (< 1 cm) are not usually detected by this technique, however, and the accuracy of CT scanning is only 40–50%. CT scanning may also be used occasionally to guide fine-needle aspiration of enlarged lymph nodes for cytological analysis to aid diagnosis.

MRI can also be used to identify metastatic disease affecting the regional lymph nodes but most scanners do not easily permit guided fine-needle aspiration. MRI may also be useful for clarifying the nature of any abnormality in equivocal bone scans and, importantly, for recognizing incipient spinal cord compression.

**PET/CT scanning.** [11]Carbon-labeled choline PET/CT and [68]gallium-labeled prostate-specific membrane antigen (PSMA) PET imaging (Figure 4.4) are accurate methods for staging advanced disease and are increasingly used to confirm or exclude the presence of soft-tissue or skeletal metastases.

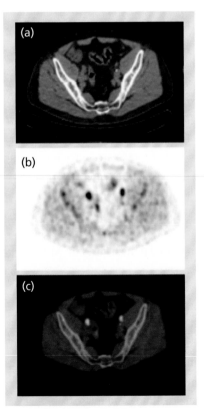

**Figure 4.4** Images from a 71-year-old patient with biopsy-proven prostate cancer. [18]F-choline PET/CT staging showed advanced disease (iliac lymph node metastases shown here). (a) CT scan, (b) PET scan and (c) PET/CT fused image. Reproduced with permission from Schwarzenböck S et al. *Theranostics* 2012;2:318–330.

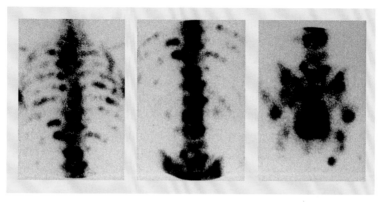

**Figure 4.5** A radionuclide bone scan showing multiple bony metastases resulting from disseminated prostate cancer.

**Radionuclide bone scanning** is reasonably sensitive for the identification of bone metastases (Figure 4.5), although false-positive findings may result from various inflammatory conditions, such as osteoarthritis. As PSA is usually a good indicator of disease progression, bone scans are not generally used to monitor disease, unless PSA or clinical factors change, especially as it can take several months for the bone scan to improve following treatment.

## Prognostic tables and nomograms

While cancer characteristics such as PSA, Gleason score, clinical stage, number of biopsy cores involved and percentage of each core involved provide valuable prognostic information, combining all these variables in a nomogram provides a much more accurate prediction of the outcome. Many of these nomograms are available on the web or as an app, such as the Memorial Sloan-Kettering Cancer Center's pretreatment nomogram (http://nomograms.mskcc.org/Prostate/PreTreatment.aspx). Nomograms are based on data from thousands of patients and are used to predict the pathological likelihood of seminal vesicle invasion, lymph node metastasis and extracapsular extension on each side, or the presence of a small, insignificant cancer. Other nomograms have been developed to predict the likelihood of recurrence of cancer after radical prostatectomy, external-beam radiotherapy or brachytherapy. Simpler prediction tools, such as

Partin's tables, predict the likely pathology from PSA values, Gleason score and clinical stage. These readily available clinical predictors are useful for patient counseling and planning treatment such as surgery or radiotherapy.

A number of tests that measure gene expression from paraffin-embedded tissue, such as prostate biopsy material, have been evaluated and appear to give prognostic information over and above that of Gleason grade grouping (see pages 14–16) alone. Three of the most developed tests are described below.

**Prolaris®** (Myriad Genetics) is a genomic 'risk stratification' test that can provide additional prognostic information to the clinical picture. It quantifies the RNA expression of 31 genes involved in tumor cell division, plus 15 'housekeeping' genes that allow standardization of the test. Low expression of these genes is associated with a low risk of cancer progression, and vice versa. The manufacturers maintain that the test can identify low- and intermediate-risk patients and those who are potentially at higher risk of cancer-specific mortality. This test can be used to counsel patients and guide therapeutic options after prostate biopsy and after radical prostatectomy.

**The Oncotype DX® prostate cancer assay** (Genomic Health) is based on the expression of multiple genes involved in androgen signaling, cellular organization, stromal response and cellular proliferation, and some housekeeping genes. A genomic prostate score allows more accurate risk stratification of patients with low -and intermediate-risk prostate cancer than is possible with the Gleason grade group alone and informs decisions about treatment.

**Decipher®** (Genomic DX Biosciences) is a gene-based test that predicts the likelihood of high-grade disease, 5-year metastasis rate and 10-year prostate cancer death based on biopsy or radical prostatectomy tissue. It can be used to decide whether a patient is suitable for active surveillance (see page 60) or whether further treatment such as radiotherapy is required in a patient with adverse pathology after radical prostatectomy.

## Summary of diagnostic and staging options

An approach to the diagnosis and staging of prostate cancer is outlined in Figure 4.6.

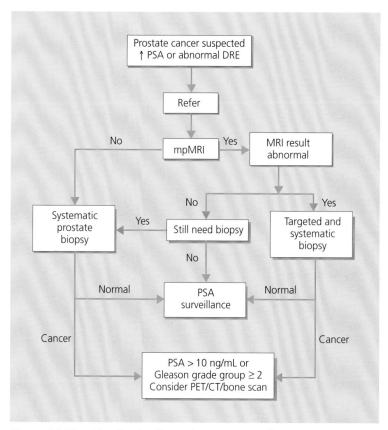

**Figure 4.6** Algorithm for the diagnosis and staging of prostate cancer. DRE, digital rectal exam; mpMRI, multiparametric magnetic resonance imaging; PSA, prostate-specific antigen.

## Key points – diagnosis, staging and prognostic indicators

- Prostate cancer is usually diagnosed on the basis of transrectal or transperineal biopsy.
- Ultrasound-guided biopsy is needed to confirm the diagnosis.
- The Gleason score of these biopsies, clinical stage on digital rectal exam (DRE) and presenting prostate-specific antigen (PSA) value provide an estimate of the risk of extraprostatic extension.
- Multiparametric MRI is increasingly used to target biopsies and can provide information about local staging.
- Bone scanning identifies bone metastases, although the probability of these in patients with PSA below 10 ng/mL is low.
- PET/CT is useful to detect soft-tissue and bone metastases.

### Key references

Afshar-Oromieh A, Haberkorn U, Eder M et al. [68Ga]Gallium-labelled PSMA ligand as superior PET tracer for the diagnosis of prostate cancer: comparison with 18F-FECH. *Eur J Nucl Med Mol Imaging* 2012;39:1085–6.

Ahmed HU, El-Shater Bosaily A, Brown LC et al; PROMIS study group. Diagnostic accuracy of multi-parametric MRI and TRUS biopsy in prostate cancer (PROMIS): a paired validating confirmatory study. *Lancet* 2017;389:815–22.

Budäus L, Leyh-Bannurah SR, Salomon G et al. Initial experience of (68)Ga-PSMA PET/CT imaging in high-risk prostate cancer patients prior to radical prostatectomy. *Eur Urol* 2016;69:393–6.

Contractor K, Challapalli A, Barwick T et al. Use of [11C]choline PET-CT as a noninvasive method for detecting pelvic lymph node status from prostate cancer and relationship with choline kinase expression. *Clin Cancer Res* 2011;17:7673–83.

de Rooij M, Crienen S, Witjes JA et al. Cost-effectiveness of magnetic resonance (MR) imaging and MR-guided targeted biopsy versus systematic transrectal ultrasound-guided biopsy in diagnosing prostate cancer: a modelling study from a health care perspective. *Eur Urol* 2014;66:430–6.

Eifler JB, Feng Z, Lin BM et al. An updated prostate cancer staging nomogram (Partin tables) based on cases from 2006 to 2011. *BJU Int* 2013;111:22–9.

Fütterer JJ, Briganti A, De Visschere P et al. Can clinically significant prostate cancer be detected with multiparametric magnetic resonance imaging? A systematic review of the literature. *Eur Urol* 2015;68: 1045–53.

Gacci M, Schiavina R, Lanciotti M et al. External validation of the updated nomogram predicting lymph node invasion in patients with prostate cancer undergoing extended pelvic lymph node dissection. *Urol Int* 2013;90:277–82.

Harisinghani MG, Barentsz J, Hahn PF et al. Noninvasive detection of clinically occult lymph-node metastases in prostate cancer. *N Engl J Med* 2003;348:2491–9.

Ishizuka O, Tanabe T, Nakayama T et al. Prostate-specific antigen, Gleason sum and clinical T stage for predicting the need for radionuclide bone scan for prostate cancer patients in Japan. *Int J Urol* 2005;12:728–32.

Iwazawa J, Mitani T, Sassa S, Ohue S. Prostate cancer detection with MRI: is dynamic contrast-enhanced imaging necessary in addition to diffusion-weighted imaging? *Diagn Interv Radiol* 2011;17:243–8.

Moore CM, Robertson NL, Arsanious N et al. Image-guided prostate biopsy using magnetic resonance imaging-derived targets: a systematic review. *Eur Urol* 2013;63:125–40.

Ohori M, Kattan MW, Koh H et al. Predicting the presence and side of extracapsular extension: a nomogram for staging prostate cancer. *J Urol* 2004;171:1844–9; discussion 1849.

Panebianco V, Barchetti F, Sciarra A et al. Multiparametric magnetic resonance imaging versus standard care in men being evaluated for prostate cancer: A randomized study. *Urol Oncol* 2015;33:17.e1–17.e7.

Patel U, Dasgupta P, Challacombe B et al. Pre-biopsy 3-Tesla MRI and targeted biopsy of the index prostate cancer: correlation with robot-assisted radical prostatectomy. *BJU Int* 2017;119:82–90.

Pokorny MR, de Rooij M, Duncan E et al. Prospective study of diagnostic accuracy comparing prostate cancer detection by transrectal ultrasound-guided biopsy versus magnetic resonance (MR) imaging with subsequent MR-guided biopsy in men without previous prostate biopsies. *Eur Urol* 2014;66:22–9.

Radkte JP, Kuru TH, Boxler S et al. Comparative analysis of transperineal template saturation prostate biopsy versus magnetic resonance imaging targeted biopsy with magnetic resonance imaging-ultrasound fusion guidance. *J Urol* 2015;193:87–94.

Schwarzenböck S, Souvatzoglou M, Krause BJ. Choline PET and PET/CT in primary diagnosis and staging of prostate cancer. *Theranostics* 2012;2:318–30.

Wegelin O, van Melick HH, Hooft L et al. Comparing three different techniques for magnetic resonance imaging-targeted prostate biopsies: a systematic review of in-bore versus magnetic resonance imaging-transrectal ultrasound fusion versus cognitive registration. Is there a preferred technique? *Eur Urol* 2017;71:517–31.

Wysock JS, Rosenkrantz AB, Huang WC et al. A prospective, blinded comparison of magnetic resonance (MR) imaging-ultrasound fusion and visual estimation in the performance of MR-targeted prostate biopsy: the PROFUS trial. *Eur Urol* 2014; 66:343–51.

Several treatment options are available for men with clinically localized prostate cancer (Table 5.1). Treatment decisions depend on many factors but the risk category is at the core. Risk groups are generally divided into very low, low, intermediate and high risk of recurrence and

TABLE 5.1

**Treatment options for localized and locally advanced prostate cancer**

| | Localized Risk of recurrence | | | Locally advanced |
|---|---|---|---|---|
| | Low | Intermediate | High | |
| Radical prostatectomy | ✓ | ✓ | ✓ | Multimodality therapy |
| EBRT | ✓ | ✓ | | |
| EBRT with androgen deprivation | | ✓ | ✓ | ✓ |
| Low-dose seed brachytherapy | ✓ | ✓ | | |
| Active surveillance | ✓ | | | |
| Watchful waiting | ✓ | ✓ | ✓ | ✓ |
| Hormonal therapy | | | ✓ | ✓ |
| *Approaches under investigation* | | | | |
| HIFU | ✓ | | | |
| Cryotherapy | ✓ | | | |

EBRT, external-beam radiotherapy; HIFU, high-intensity focused ultrasonography.

are based on Gleason grade group (see pages 14–16), number of biopsy cores involved, prostate-specific antigen (PSA) level and clinical stage (Table 5.2). Unfortunately, our current knowledge is such that it is not always possible to predict which treatments will produce the optimum outcome for an individual, so patient choice is an important factor. It may be possible to build a prognostic picture using genetic markers of cell cycle progression. Promising results with the Prolaris genomic test (see page 54) suggest that it may add prognostic value to current methods. Other gene-based tests such as Oncotype DX and Decipher (see page 54) also offer considerable potential.

The aim in treating localized prostate cancer of significant grade and tumor volume is usually curative if the man has a reasonable life expectancy, or prevention of death *from* prostate cancer (as opposed to death *with* prostate cancer) in men with shorter life expectancy. The likelihood of a man with localized prostate cancer dying from the disease itself, as opposed to other causes, increases with the risk category but decreases with age and comorbidities. As men with localized disease often do not experience significant disease-related morbidity for many years after diagnosis, and curative treatment itself may result in some morbidity, those with lower-risk cancers and a shorter life expectancy are least likely to benefit from radical treatment.

## Active surveillance

Active surveillance is increasingly popular, particularly for men with small-volume and low-to-moderate-grade prostate cancer (very-low- or low-risk category), who have a low risk of death from prostate cancer (Table 5.3). These men are eligible for curative therapy but this option is often deferred until objective signs of disease progression are observed. This approach means that the majority of men (60–70%) are spared the side effects of curative therapy that they do not require. Recent studies have shown that men with low-risk prostate cancer have a low risk of developing metastases, although the risk is reasonably high for men with intermediate-risk cancers. Therefore, younger men with intermediate risk cancers should usually be encouraged to choose treatment rather than active surveillance.

TABLE 5.2

**Categories of risk of recurrence**

| Risk category | TNM stage | Gleason grade group | PSA (ng/mL) | Biopsy results* | PSA density (ng/mL/g) |
|---|---|---|---|---|---|
| Very low | T1c | 1 | < 10 | < 3 +ve/ < 50% | < 0.15 |
| Low | T1–T2 | 1 | < 10 | | |
| Intermediate | T2b–T2c, *or* | 2 or 3 | 10–20 | | |
| High | T3a, *or* | 4 or 5 | > 20 | | |

*Positive biopsy cores/cancer in each core.
PSA, prostate-specific antigen; TNM, tumor–nodes–metastasis.
National Comprehensive Cancer Network (NCCN) guidelines, 2017.

TABLE 5.3

**Active surveillance criteria**

**Consider men with:**

- PSA < 15 ng/mL
- Gleason biopsy score ≤ 3 + 3
- Low volume < 4 mm of any core, and ≤ 3/12 cores involved
- Life expectancy > 10 years/suitable for radical treatment of progression

**Confirming:**

- 3-Tesla multiparametric MRI showing no index or significant lesion
- Repeat TRUS or transperineal biopsy (if available) within first 6–12 months shows no upgrading or increased volume of cancer

**Radical treatment indicated by:**

- PSA velocity > 1 ng/mL/year
- Clinical progression on DRE
- Increase in Gleason score on repeat biopsy
- Patient choice

DRE, digital rectal exam; MRI, magnetic resonance imaging; PSA, prostate-specific antigen; TRUS, transrectal ultrasonography.

Active surveillance involves PSA measurement and a digital rectal exam (DRE) every 3–6 months. MRI and repeat biopsies are usually organized 6–12 months after diagnosis or if cancer progression is suspected. Increasingly, multiparametric MRI (see page 45) is also being used to select patients for entry or follow-up in active surveillance protocols. Curative-intent therapy is initiated if the cancer shows signs of progression and before it becomes incurable. Cancer-specific survival in men who fit the criteria for active surveillance is 99% at 8 years' follow-up. While men avoid the physical side effects of treatment, they do have to live with the psychological effects of having an untreated cancer, although these do not seem to be troublesome for most men. In most untreated series, only about one-third of men managed by active surveillance progressed to active treatment, and those who did were usually cured.

## Radical prostatectomy

Radical prostatectomy involves surgical removal of the entire prostate and seminal vesicles and a variable amount of adjacent tissue (Figure 5.1), and is appropriate if it is believed that the tumor can be removed completely, and where the patient satisfies the criteria set out in Table 5.4. The procedure used to be commonly performed via the retropubic route but it is now increasingly performed laparoscopically with robotic assistance. A perineal approach is also possible but this has fallen out of favor.

The major advantage of radical prostatectomy is that all prostatic tissue is excised and it provides precise histological information and definitive cure in patients in whom the tumor is confined to the prostate, relieving the patient's anxiety. Given that prostate cancer has a long natural history, this is an important consideration in terms of the patient's quality of life. Long-term studies have shown normal life expectancy in patients with complete excision of specimen-confined disease. Ten-year survival for men with clinically localized disease treated with radical prostatectomy is 98% for Gleason grade group 1, and 91% and 76% for groups 2–3 and 4–5, respectively. Moreover, the procedure also offers definitive treatment of concomitant benign prostatic hyperplasia (BPH) and associated lower urinary tract

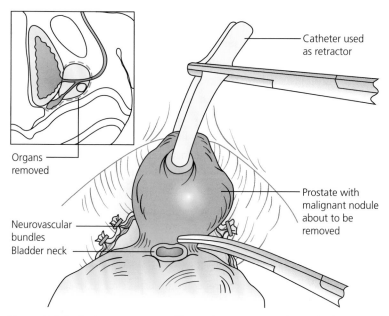

Catheter used
as retractor

Organs
removed

Prostate with
malignant nodule
about to be
removed

Neurovascular
bundles
Bladder neck

**Figure 5.1** Radical prostatectomy. The entire prostate and attached seminal vesicles are removed and an anastomosis created between the bladder neck and the urethra.

TABLE 5.4

**Selection criteria for radical prostatectomy**

- Histological evidence of prostate cancer
- Clinically localized disease (stages T1–T2)
- Life expectancy > 10 years
- No contraindications to surgery
- No significant comorbidity

symptoms and reliably results in undetectable PSA, which patients find reassuring.

The principal adverse events associated with radical prostatectomy are (usually mild) stress urinary incontinence (< 2–3%) and erectile dysfunction (> 50%); the latter is age related, tends to improve with time and can be minimized by nerve-sparing approaches. Moreover, erectile dysfunction after surgery can now be treated quite effectively (see Chapter 9). Table 5.5 summarizes the advantages and disadvantages of radical prostatectomy.

Most urologists believe that radical prostatectomy, however achieved, offers the best opportunity for complete and permanent cure in patients with localized prostate cancer. A randomized study from Sweden showed that, at a median follow-up of 8.2 years, radical prostatectomy decreased prostate-cancer-related mortality by 44% and overall death by 26% when compared with watchful waiting. The difference was greatest in men under 65 years of age. Because the total number of prostate-cancer-related deaths was low, the number needed to treat (NNT) to save one death was 20.

A similar US study, the Prostate Cancer Intervention Versus Observation Trial (PIVOT), which had a high proportion of patients with low-risk prostate cancer, reported no difference in overall survival (OS) at a median follow-up of 10 years, but radical prostatectomy in men with high-risk cancers provided a 60% reduction in prostate

TABLE 5.5

**Advantages and disadvantages of treatment options for localized prostate cancer**

### Radical prostatectomy

| Advantages | Disadvantages |
|---|---|
| • High likelihood of cure if tumor pathologically confined | • Major operation |
| | • Potential mortality ($< 0.4\%$) |
| • Definitive staging possible | • Potential morbidity: |
| • Treatment of concomitant BPH | – Erectile dysfunction ($> 50\%$) |
| • Reliable PSA suppression to unrecordable levels | – Persistent incontinence ($< 3\%$) |
| • Side effects improve with time | – Pulmonary embolism ($< 1\%$) |
| • Easy monitoring for recurrent disease | – Bladder neck stricture ($< 5\%$) |
| | – Infertility |
| • Radiotherapy possible after surgery | CONTINUED |

TABLE 5.5 (CONTINUED)

## Advantages and disadvantages of treatment options for localized prostate cancer

### Radiotherapy

| *Advantages* | *Disadvantages* |
|---|---|
| • Potential cure | • Prostate left in situ |
| • Surgery avoided | • Difficulty assessing cure |
| • Outpatient therapy | • No definitive staging possible |
| | • No benefit for concomitant BPH |
| | • Patient anxiety during follow-up |
| | • Unreliable PSA suppression |
| | • May need concomitant ADT |
| | • Potential morbidity: |
| |   – Rectal injury (2–10%) |
| |   – Urinary incontinence (< 3%) |
| |   – Impotence (20–30%) |
| |   – Bladder damage (10–20%) |
| |   – Hematuria (5–10%) |
| | • Surgery has a greater morbidity after radiotherapy |

### Brachytherapy

| *Advantages* | *Disadvantages* |
|---|---|
| • One-off treatment | • Only appropriate for low-risk disease |
| • Day-case or overnight procedure | • Cannot be used after previous prostate surgery |
| • Limited period of catheterization | • Limited experience of long-term effects |
| • Low risk of incontinence | • Difficulty assessing cure |
| • Lower risk of erectile dysfunction | • Makes subsequent surgery dangerous |
| | • Significant urinary symptoms in first 6 months |

ADT, androgen deprivation therapy; BPH, benign prostatic hyperplasia; PSA, prostate-specific antigen.

cancer mortality. However, the trial has been criticized for under-recruitment and inclusion of many men with significant comorbidities, leading to an excessive death rate from non-prostate-related causes.

The most recent study, ProtecT, randomized men with predominantly low- and intermediate-risk cancers to active surveillance, radical prostatectomy or radiotherapy. The outcomes at 10 years showed no difference in mortality between surgery and radiotherapy, while those on active surveillance had a substantially greater risk (almost double) of developing metastases than those who underwent active treatment. This study has been criticized on the basis of the allocation of intermediate-risk patients to active surveillance, and because a difference in mortality between surgery and radiotherapy would not be expected as early as 10 years in men with predominantly low/intermediate-risk disease.

Surgery can also be effective for high-risk prostate cancer, particularly if the disease appears to be localized to the prostate gland. In cases of T3 prostate cancer, surgery may be appropriate if it is considered that the cancer can be fully excised. A multimodal approach that includes adjuvant radiotherapy should be considered. Following surgery, patients who have adverse pathological features such as extracapsular extension, seminal vesicle extension or positive margins can be treated with adjuvant radiotherapy to the prostatic bed, often with concomitant androgen ablation (see pages 86–90). Three randomized trials have shown that this decreases the risk of PSA recurrence by 52% compared with no treatment, and improves survival. Whether early salvage radiation is equivalent to adjuvant radiation is not yet known, and salvage radiotherapy remains an option in these patients (see Chapter 6).

Extended lymph node dissection should also be considered in men undergoing radical prostatectomy for high-risk cancer. This strategy more accurately stages the tumor, allowing for better prognostication and institution of adjuvant therapies; whether it improves recurrence rates and survival is yet to be proven.

**Neoadjuvant hormonal therapy prior to radical prostatectomy** has been shown to reduce PSA levels, prostate volume and tumor volume, and decreases positive surgical margins. However, advantages in terms of cancer recurrence or survival have not been demonstrated so this practice remains investigational.

**Robotic-assisted radical prostatectomy** (Figure 5.2) has become the technique of choice in most centers. It provides similar oncological outcomes to open radical prostatectomy, based on recent systematic reviews and meta-analysis, but recovery of urinary incontinence and erectile function at 12 months is probably marginally better after robotic-assisted surgery. The operating time is somewhat longer, but blood loss and length of hospital stay are significantly reduced, and recovery is quicker; patients also return to work sooner. The ten-times greater magnification and more-precise instrumentation with robotic-assisted radical prostatectomy contribute to these differences, and robotic assistance certainly makes the surgery easier to perform.

A recent randomized study that compared outcomes with open and robotic-assisted radical prostatectomy found no substantial differences

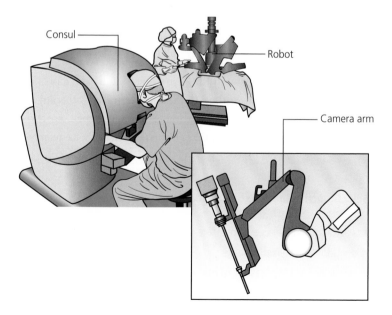

**Figure 5.2** Robotic-assisted radical prostatectomy using the da Vinci surgical system.

in incontinence, erectile function and positive margins at 3 months. Open prostatectomy was associated with higher rates of complications and transfusion. This study has been criticized for comparing a surgeon who was experienced in open surgery versus a less-experienced robotic surgeon, and the follow-up was short.

## Radiotherapy

**External-beam radiotherapy** (EBRT) is widely used in the treatment of localized and locally advanced prostate cancer, offering a particular advantage in patients who are unsuitable for surgery because of comorbidity or evidence of extraprostatic spread of the cancer. The eligibility criteria for radiotherapy are shown in Table 5.6. Standard treatment generally involves an 8-week course of three-dimensional conformal radiotherapy, or intensity-modulated radiotherapy (IMRT) delivering at at least 78 Gy. The recently completed CHHiP trial (Conventional or Hypofractionated High Dose Intensity Modulated Radiotherapy for Prostate Cancer) showed that hypofractionation can decrease the duration of radiotherapy delivery to 4 weeks but with no difference in cancer recurrence rates or side effects; however, this study has been criticized for undertreating the control arm with only 74 Gy.

The principal side effects with EBRT are due to radiation damage to the bladder, urethra and rectum. In the short term, radiotherapy to the prostate causes frequency of urination, dysuria, diarrhea, proctitis and tiredness. In the longer term, there is a risk of urinary frequency

TABLE 5.6

**Selection criteria for external-beam radiotherapy**

- Histological evidence of prostate cancer
- Regionally localized disease
- Sufficient life expectancy to make cure potentially beneficial
- Absence of lower urinary tract disorders (particularly outflow obstruction)
- Absence of colorectal disease

and bleeding, which may be severe in 2–3% of patients. Rectal side effects consist of urgency, frequency, tenesmus and bleeding. Erectile dysfunction due to damage to the neurovascular supply to the corpora cavernosa can also occur, often gradually over a 6–18-month period. In the longer term there is an increased risk of rectal and bladder cancers.

Recent advances in the delivery of radiotherapy include image-guided radiotherapy, in which gold seed 'fiducial' markers are placed within the prostate to focus the radiotherapy beams more accurately, increasing radiation delivery to the target and reducing damage to surrounding structures.

A number of studies have shown that cancer control is better in men with intermediate- or high-risk prostate cancer if the radiation dose is escalated beyond 78 Gy. IMRT allows precise targeting of the prostate, with less radiation scatter to surrounding organs, allowing higher doses of radiation to be used without a significant increase in local toxicity. The advantages and disadvantages of radiotherapy are summarized in Table 5.5 and are compared with those of radical prostatectomy and brachytherapy.

External-beam radiation alone (i.e. without prior hormonal reduction therapy) is no longer recommended, particularly for patients with intermediate- or high-risk disease. Prior reduction of the tumor burden using a luteinizing hormone-releasing hormone (LHRH) analog/antagonist (see pages 88–9) or an antiandrogen (see pages 89–90) appears to increase the sensitivity of cancer cells to irradiation. This approach has been validated in randomized trials, which showed that both progression-free survival and OS were significantly improved when men with high-risk prostate cancers were treated with adjuvant hormonal therapy and EBRT. In one US trial, the addition of concomitant androgen deprivation therapy to radiotherapy improved the 10-year OS rate from 39.8% to 58.1% and reduced the 10-year prostate cancer mortality rate from 30.4% to 10.3% (Figure 5.3). Similar improvements have been noted in other North American trials. It is now standard practice for men undergoing EBRT for high-risk disease to also receive pretreatment hormonal therapy, and this is often continued for a variable time after treatment.

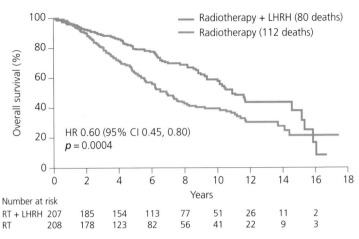

**Figure 5.3** In a randomized trial involving men at high risk of developing metastases, the addition of an LHRH agonist during external-beam radiotherapy and for 3 years after improved 10-year overall survival. CI, confidence interval; HR, hazard ratio. Reproduced from Bolla et al. *Lancet Oncol* 2010;11:1066–73, with permission from Elsevier.

**CyberKnife** stereotactic body radiation therapy uses computer-assisted image guidance to target about 1200 beams of high-energy radiation to the tumor (Figure 5.4). It can correct for prostate movement, which helps to reduce irradiation of surrounding tissue. Evidence is building to support its use in men with early localized prostate cancer, and early data suggest a role in men with intermediate-risk cancer. Patients tend to appreciate the short duration of treatment (usually only a week). However, longer-term follow-up data are required before CyberKnife becomes an established treatment.

**Proton beam therapy** differs from standard photon-based radiation therapy in that the penetration of the heavy, charged protons is limited because of low energy, minimizing damage to surrounding structures and allowing dose escalation. Most published studies have not shown any substantial difference in cancer outcomes between IMRT and proton beam therapy and, interestingly, proton beam therapy has been associated with equivalent or even greater toxicity. Proton beam therapy is expensive, and in the absence of any obvious advantage in

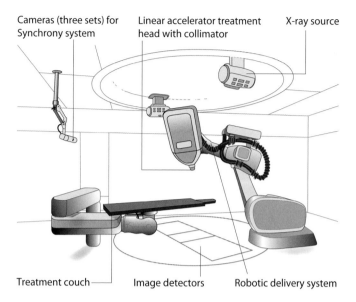

Cameras (three sets) for Synchrony system

Linear accelerator treatment head with collimator

X-ray source

Treatment couch

Image detectors

Robotic delivery system

**Figure 5.4** The CyberKnife treatment delivery system. Powerful imaging aids accurate targeting of high-energy radiation to the tumor.

cancer control or toxicity, most radiation oncologists prefer tried and tested IMRT for prostate cancer.

**Low-dose seed brachytherapy** involves careful placing of either iodine-125 or palladium-103 seeds into the prostate via the transperineal route, using a grid template and transrectal ultrasonography (TRUS) guidance (see Figure 4.3, page 49). Patient selection criteria are given in Table 5.7. The results of seed brachytherapy in men with low-risk disease (PSA < 10 ng/mL, Gleason score < 7, ≤ cT2b) are equivalent to those of radical prostatectomy at 10 years but are highly dependent on the quality of seed placement. The results in patients with intermediate risk are worse, however, with approximately 66% of men free from recurrence at 10 years.

This technique is popular, particularly in the USA, because of its low morbidity; the side effects are similar to those of external-beam radiotherapy but may also include difficulty with urination because of prostate swelling. In general, brachytherapy is not suitable if the prostate volume is much greater than 50 cm$^3$ or for men with severe

TABLE 5.7

**Selection criteria for low-dose seed brachytherapy**

- Histological evidence of prostate cancer
- Clinically localized disease (T1 or T2)
- Low PSA (preferably < 10 ng/mL)
- Low–moderate Gleason score (6 or 7) preferable
- Prostate volume not large (< 50 cm³)
- Minimal obstructive urinary symptoms
- No prior transurethral resection of the prostate

pre-existing bladder outflow obstruction. Previous transurethral resection of the prostate (TURP) is usually also a contraindication to brachytherapy because it can be difficult to place the seeds accurately. Although salvage therapy after brachytherapy is possible, the risks of surgery are considerably greater than in de novo cases.

## Watchful waiting

Watchful waiting is different from active surveillance – it is for men who are older or have shorter life expectancy, and for those who have prostate cancer that is unlikely to shorten life. These men are counseled and reviewed regularly with clinical examination and PSA measurements. If disease progression is identified, palliative androgen deprivation is initiated and continued until death, rather than instigating curative therapy. In a recent meta-analysis, the development of metastatic disease during watchful waiting was 2.1% per year in patients with well-differentiated tumors (Gleason scores 2–4), compared with 13.5% per year in patients with aggressive tumors (Gleason scores 7–10). In another study, patients with low-grade tumors who underwent watchful waiting had a 92% disease-specific survival at 10 years, compared with 76% for moderate-grade tumors and 43% for high-grade tumors.

Men with high-risk prostate cancer have a considerably increased risk of prostate cancer-specific mortality. However, if significant comorbidities are present, watchful waiting may still be the most appropriate treatment option, given that they are more likely to succumb to other comorbid conditions. Patients and their immediate family should be fully informed about the implications of opting for watchful waiting; PSA values should be monitored regularly, and timely symptomatic treatment offered as appropriate.

## Experimental techniques

**High-intensity focused ultrasonography** (HIFU) has been developed for the treatment of localized prostate cancer. A probe delivers HIFU transrectally to the prostate and achieves focal tissue destruction. Early results are promising, with some series reporting that about three-quarters of men with low-risk disease are disease free at 5 years' follow-up. HIFU can also be used for the treatment of cancer recurrence after radiotherapy. This technique should currently be regarded as experimental, particularly as the side effects of incontinence and the development of a urinary fistula may be troublesome and are often difficult to resolve. The reliability and durability of this treatment is still uncertain.

**Cryoablation.** Under TRUS guidance, cryogenic probes are inserted into the prostate via the perineum and liquid nitrogen is circulated through the probes, producing 'ice balls' with a temperature of approximately −180°C that disrupt cell membranes, thereby destroying the surrounding tissue. The urethra is protected by circulating warm water (44°C) through a catheter. Although some studies have reported that outcomes are similar to those with radical prostatectomy, others have reported a significant incidence of complications, such as rectal and urethral damage and occasional fistula formation. Cryoablation has yet to be compared with more established treatments in long-term randomized controlled trials, and the treatment may be more applicable to patients with recurrence after radiotherapy, although formation of prostatorectal and vescicorectal fistulas remains a problem.

**MRI–ultrasound fusion-targeted cryotherapy.** A recent small study in men with intermediate- and high-risk prostate cancer demonstrated the feasibility of MRI–TRUS fusion (see page 48) focal cryotherapy in the majority of patients, and accurately guided ablation, as demonstrated by post-treatment imaging, with little genitourinary toxicity. Additional studies are needed to determine the efficacy of this approach using post-cryotherapy biopsy.

**Vascular-targeted photodynamic therapy** (VTP) is a new treatment developed in Israel; it involves injecting a padeliporfin, a light-sensitive drug developed from deep-sea seaweed, into the bloodstream and activating it using a laser fiber introduced transperineally, destroying tumor tissue whilst preserving the normal prostate tissue. Early results are encouraging but this technique is not yet used in the clinic. About half of the patients (49%) treated with VTP went into complete remission, compared with 13.5% in the control group (who were managed by active surveillance). Further trials are needed to confirm these findings, and it may therefore be several years until this technique becomes widely available.

### Antiandrogen monotherapy

Hormonal therapy is discussed in full in Chapter 7. Conventional hormone ablation therapy for locally advanced prostate cancer (T3 or T4) involves the use of depot LHRH analogs, preceded and accompanied by an antiandrogen for at least 2–6 weeks and sometimes continued thereafter for up to 3 years. Randomized trials have shown that monotherapy with the antiandrogen bicalutamide, 150 mg/day, is as effective in the control of locally advanced disease as castration by either orchidectomy or an LHRH analog. In addition, a very large international randomized trial, with median follow-up of 7.4 years, showed that adjuvant treatment with bicalutamide, 150 mg/ day, plus standard therapy for locally advanced prostate cancer (i.e. surgery, radiotherapy or watchful waiting) significantly reduced objective progression by 31% when compared with standard therapy. A survival benefit of 35% was also observed in men receiving radiation with adjuvant bicalutamide.

Use of an antiandrogen has the advantage of potentially preserving libido and sexual function (Figure 5.5). Younger patients often opt for

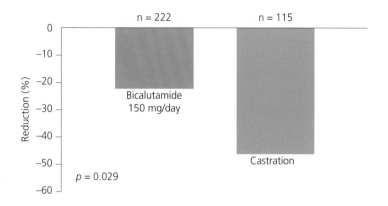

**Figure 5.5** Reduction from baseline in sexual interest after 12 months' treatment with bicalutamide, 150 mg/day, or castration (surgical or chemical) in patients with M0 prostate cancer. Adapted from Iversen P. 1999.

treatment that has less impact on this important aspect of their lives but they should be warned that gynecomastia is likely. If progression occurs, treatment with an LHRH analog may prove beneficial.

## Management of local complications

Locally advanced prostate cancer may cause any of several urologic emergencies. Acute or chronic urinary retention may require TURP. Care should be taken with this procedure not to induce stress or complete urinary incontinence, because the normal landmarks can be distorted by the tumor. A period of catheter drainage during androgen ablation, followed by a trial without the catheter, is often indicated before surgery.

Anuria resulting from bilateral ureteric obstruction, due to enlarged lymph nodes at the vesico–ureteric junction or pelvic brim, may necessitate insertion of nephrostomy tubes or passage of a double-pigtail stent and subsequent EBRT. Pelvic lymphadenopathy can also cause unilateral or bilateral leg swelling due to compression of the iliac veins, occasionally requiring venous stenting.

Bleeding from the tumor may occasionally precipitate hematuria and clot retention, requiring bladder washout and irrigation and, sometimes, diathermy – or even embolization – of bleeding tumor vessels.

**Key points – management of clinically localized disease**

- The treatment of localized prostate cancer is controversial.
- Active surveillance is increasingly used for very-low- and low-risk disease.
- Only about one-third of men managed with active surveillance will go on to require curative treatment.
- Radical prostatectomy probably offers the best prospect of long-term cure but carries the disadvantages of possible sexual dysfunction and incontinence.
- In the case of high-risk cancer, surgery may be considered as part of a multimodal therapeutic approach.
- External-beam radiotherapy (EBRT) can be curative but may be associated with rectal or bladder complications.
- Brachytherapy can be combined with EBRT in higher-risk individuals.
- Treatment with EBRT and hormonal therapy is more effective than radiotherapy alone in men with intermediate- and high-risk cancer.
- In a large international trial, the antiandrogen bicalutamide, 150 mg/day, reduced objective progression by 31% but gynecomastia was common.

# Key references

Albertsen PC, Hanley JA, Fine J. 20-year outcomes following conservative management of clinically localized prostate cancer. *JAMA* 2005;293:2095–101.

Azzouzi AR, Vincendeau S, Barret E et al.; PCM301 Study Group. Padeliporfin vascular-targeted photodynamic therapy versus active surveillance in men with low-risk prostate cancer (CLIN1001 PCM301): an open-label, phase 3, randomised controlled trial. *Lancet Oncol* 2017;18:181–91.

Bill-Axelson A, Holmberg L, Ruutu M et al. Radical prostatectomy versus watchful waiting in early prostate cancer. *N Engl J Med* 2005;352:1977–84.

Bolla M, Van Tienhoven G, Warde P et al. External irradiation with or without long-term androgen suppression for prostate cancer with high metastatic risk: 10-year results of an EORTC randomised study. *Lancet Oncol* 2010;11:1066–73.

D'Amico AV, Chen MH, Renshaw AA et al. Androgen suppression and radiation vs radiation alone for prostate cancer: a randomized trial. *JAMA* 2008;299:289–95.

D'Amico AV, Denham JW, Bolla M et al. Short- vs long-term androgen suppression plus external beam radiation therapy and survival in men of advanced age with node-negative high-risk adenocarcinoma of the prostate. *Cancer* 2007;109:2004–10.

Dearnaley D, Syndikus I, Mossop H et al.; on behalf of the CHHiP Investigators. Conventional versus hypofractionated high-dose intensity-modulated radiotherapy for prostate cancer: 5-year outcomes of the randomised, non-inferiority, phase 3 CHHiP trial. *Lancet Oncol* 2016;17:1047–60.

Hamdy FC, Donovan JL, Lane JA et al. for the ProtecT study group. 10-year outcomes after monitoring, surgery, or radiotherapy for localized prostate cancer. *N Engl J Med* 2016;375:1415–24.

Iversen P. Quality of life issues relating to endocrine treatment options. Eur Urol 1999;36 Suppl 2:20–6.

Klotz L, Vespirini D, Sethukavalan P et al. Long-term follow-up of a large active surveillance cohort of patients with prostate cancer. *J Clin Oncol* 2015;33:272–7.

Lane A, Metcalfe C, Young GJ et al.; ProtecT Study group. Patient-reported outcomes in the ProtecT randomized trial of clinically localized prostate cancer treatments: study design, and baseline urinary, bowel and sexual function and quality of life. *BJU Int* 2016; 118:869–79.

Thompson IM, Tangen CM, Paradelo J et al. Adjuvant radiotherapy for pathological T3N0M0 prostate cancer significantly reduces risk of metastases and improves survival: long-term followup of a randomized clinical trial. *J Urol* 2009;181: 956–62.

Uchida T, Ohkusa H, Yamashita H et al. Five years experience of transrectal high-intensity focused ultrasound using the Sonablate device in the treatment of localized prostate cancer. *Int J Urol* 2006;13:228–33.

Valerio M, Shah TT, Shah P et al. Magnetic resonance imaging-transrectal ultrasound fusion focal cryotherapy of the prostate: a prospective development study. *Urol Oncol* 2016 Dec 7. pii: S1078-1439(16)30374-X. doi: 10.1016/j.urolonc.2016.11.008. [Epub ahead of print].

Wilt TJ, Brawer MK, Jones KM et al. Radical prostatectomy versus observation for localized prostate cancer. *N Engl J Med* 2012;367: 203–13.

Yamamoto T, Musunuru B, Vesprini D et al. Metastatic prostate cancer in men initially treated with active surveillance. *J Urol* 2016;195: 1409–14.

Recurrence after initial surgery or radiotherapy usually manifests as a rise in serum prostate-specific antigen (PSA). Digital rectal exam (DRE), CT or MRI, and bone scan are the next steps but may not reveal a specific site unless the PSA level is significantly raised. A prostate-specific membrane antigen (PSMA) PET scan (see page 52) may reveal sites of cancer recurrence at very low PSA levels, typically in the prostate bed (after prostatectomy), within the prostate (after radiotherapy) or in more distant lymph nodes or bone sites. Less commonly, pulmonary metastases may be detected. The likelihood of having a positive PSMA PET scan at various PSA levels is shown in Figure 6.1. If the site of recurrence can be identified, appropriate therapy can then be delivered.

## Recurrence after prostatectomy

Prostate cancer recurs in 15–46% of men who undergo radical prostatectomy. Risk factors for recurrence include:

- positive surgical margins
- extracapsular extension
- seminal vesicle involvement

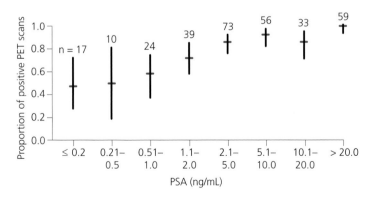

**Figure 6.1.** Incidence of positive PET scan according to level of prostate-specific antigen (PSA). Adapted from Afshar-Oromieh A et al. 2015.

- lymph node metastases at the time of surgery
- higher-grade cancer (Gleason score $\geq$ 8).

The PSA level should reliably fall to below 0.1 ng/mL after prostatectomy. The recommendations for cut-off values that indicate cancer recurrence range from 0.2 to 0.5 ng/mL. If the PSA level does not fall below this level within 6 weeks of surgery, systemic disease should be suspected.

Cancer recurrence is confirmed if the PSA level is above the cut-off and rising with sequential measurements, but time to metastasis and death is variable and is often quite prolonged. On average, a patient with recurrence of raised PSA will develop metastases over a median of 8 years, with death 5 years after the development of metastases. A number of factors determine how fast the cancer recurrence actually progresses:

- time to recurrence after prostatectomy – a shorter time to recurrence is associated with faster disease progression
- doubling of the PSA level in less than 3 months is associated with shorter time to metastases and death
- higher Gleason grade group is associated with faster progression (see pages 14–16).

When only a raised PSA level is seen, it is not known whether the recurrence is local (in the prostate bed) or systemic (metastases). In the absence of a PSMA PET scan, several factors can also help with estimation of the likelihood of local versus systemic disease (Table 6.1).

A number of choices are available for the management of PSA recurrence, including watchful waiting, salvage radiotherapy and hormonal therapy.

**Watchful waiting** is ideal for a man with a limited life expectancy and/or lower probability of disease progression based on the earlier criteria. It should be remembered that, in the average patient, metastases do not develop until 8 years after a PSA rise is detected, with death 5 years later. This treatment can be offered to men who have recurrence in the prostate bed or at distant metastatic sites confirmed by PSMA PET.

TABLE 6.1

**PSA and pathological features that predict local or systemic recurrence following radical prostatectomy**

|  | Local recurrence | Systemic recurrence |
|---|---|---|
| Gleason score | ≤ 7 | > 7 |
| Lymph node invasion | No | Yes |
| PSA doubling time | > 12 months | < 3 months |
| Seminal vesicle involvement | No | Yes |
| Time to PSA recurrence | > 1 year | < 1 year |

**Salvage radiotherapy** is a potentially curative treatment for men with a high likelihood of residual cancer in the prostatic bed. The best results are in men who have a Gleason grade group of 3 or lower, pre-radiotherapy PSA below 1.0 ng/mL, positive surgical margins, and a PSA doubling time of more than 10 months. It is also more effective if PSMA PET confirms that the prostate bed is the only site of recurrence. The effectiveness of salvage radiation is improving, with 60–90% of men achieving undetectable PSA levels, especially if concomitant androgen ablation is used (see page 86–90).

Side effects include possible loss of erectile function, bladder neck contracture and radiation proctitis. Androgen ablation with an antiandrogen or luteinizing hormone-releasing hormone (LHRH) analog/antagonist is increasingly used to enhance the effectiveness of the radiation treatment and can continue for 12–24 months.

**Hormonal therapy** is reserved for men who have progressive PSA rises and are unlikely to harbor isolated local recurrence, or have confirmed widespread metastatic disease. The timing for initiation of hormonal therapy in these men is controversial, however. A recent randomized trial has shown that immediate hormonal therapy for PSA recurrence resulted in better overall survival (OS) than delayed treatment. Hormone therapy is described in greater detail in Chapter 7.

## Recurrence following radiation therapy

The definition of recurrence is less straightforward after radiation treatment than after surgery, and the natural history of PSA recurrence is less clear after radiation than surgery. Following radiation, the PSA level falls slowly over 12–24 months to a nadir at detectable levels, usually below 1.0 ng/mL. However, approximately 30% of men have a transient rise (a 'bounce') in the first 2 years, and, complicating matters further, adjuvant hormonal therapy is often used, which suppresses PSA, although once this is stopped, the PSA slowly rises as the testosterone levels rise.

Currently, recurrence after radiation therapy is defined as a PSA level that is 2 ng/mL or more above the nadir level. PSA doubling time (see page 80) is usually the best predictor of metastatic disease; a PSA doubling time of less than 3 months is associated with a higher risk of death.

Once PSA recurrence has been identified, further investigations depend on the individual's circumstances and expectations, and involve determining whether the cancer is in the prostate, systemic or both. PSMA PET can be used in addition to staging CT/MRI and bone scan. A prostate re-biopsy can be performed if salvage treatment for local disease is being considered, although tissue sampling is often more difficult because of post-radiation fibrosis, and the result is often negative. There are several options for treatment.

- Watchful waiting can be offered to men who have limited life expectancy, and/or progression of the cancer is slow.
- Salvage prostatectomy is an option if the tumor is likely to be limited to the prostate; however, it is considerably more difficult than in men who have not received radiotherapy and has a significantly higher incidence of side effects, particularly stress incontinence.
- Cryotherapy and high-intensity focused ultrasonography (HIFU) (see page 73) are also options but also carry significant risks of complications.
- Hormonal therapy is usually reserved for men who do not have isolated localized disease. As when following prostatectomy, hormone therapy for recurrence after radiation therapy improves survival if given early.

**Oligometastatic disease.** The advent of PSMA and choline PET scans has allowed earlier and more precise identification of metastases. Disease is described as oligometastatic when metastases are limited (3–5). This disease probably incorporates a spectrum of biologies, ranging from cancers that will soon become widespread metastases to those that will remain relatively indolent. A number of studies have reported on the treatment of oligometastatic lesions by surgical removal (salvage lymph node dissection) or, more often, stereotactic radiotherapy. While the results have been somewhat conflicting, only a small proportion of men gain long-term freedom from progression with these salvage therapies.

The TROG 03.04 randomized controlled trial in men with locally advanced prostate cancer sought to determine whether eradication of oligometastases by stereotactic body radiation therapy (i.e. CyberKnife) (or other means) can result in cure or prolongation of survival in some cases (rather than solely providing palliation) using risk–survival models. A clear prognostic gradient based on the number of sites of bony metastases was identified, and further bony metastatic progression in men with up to three bony metastases had a major impact on prostate cancer-specific mortality. Bone progression made a greater contribution to prostate cancer-specific mortality than progression at other sites.

**Key points – managing recurrence after initial therapy**

- Prostate-specific antigen (PSA) level should reliably fall to below 0.1 ng/mL following radical prostatectomy.
- Recurrence after prostatectomy is generally defined as PSA above 0.2 ng/mL and rising.
- Recurrence after radiation therapy is usually defined as PSA that is at least 2 ng/mL above the nadir.
- For the average patient, metastases do not develop until 8 years after a PSA rise is detected, with death some 5 years later, so watchful waiting is an appropriate option for some men with recurrence.
- Prostate-specific membrane antigen (PSMA) PET/CT can be used to evaluate men who have a PSA rise after local treatment.
- Following prostatectomy, patients who have a high likelihood of local disease can be offered salvage radiotherapy.
- Following radiotherapy, patients who have recurrence in the prostate only may be offered a salvage treatment such as radical prostatectomy, High-intensity focused ultrasonography (HIFU) or cryotherapy, but all of these carry the risk of side effects.
- Progressive PSA rises following initial therapy suggest micrometastatic disease, which should be treated with hormone therapy; however, the timing of this treatment is controversial.
- More evidence is needed from clinical trials to inform us of the most effective treatment options in these situations.

## Key references

Afshar-Oromieh A, Avtzi E, Giesel FL et al. The diagnostic value of PET/CT imaging with the (68)Ga-labelled PSMA ligand HBED-CC in the diagnosis of recurrent prostate cancer. *Eur J Nucl Med Mol Imaging* 2015;42:197–209.

Chade DC, Eastham J, Graefen M et al. Cancer control and functional outcomes of salvage radical prostatectomy for radiation-recurrent prostate cancer: a systematic review of the literature. *Eur Urol* 2012;61:961–71.

D'Amico AV, Moul J, Carroll PR et al. Prostate specific antigen doubling time as a surrogate end point for prostate cancer specific mortality following radical prostatectomy or radiation therapy. *J Urol* 2004;172:S42–6.

Duchesne GM, Woo HH, Bassett JK et al. Timing of androgen-deprivation therapy in patients with prostate cancer with a rising PSA (TROG 03.06 and VCOG PR 01-03 [TOAD]): a randomised, multicentre, non-blinded, phase 3 trial. *Lancet Oncol* 2016;17:727–37.

Freedland SJ, Humphreys EB, Mangold LA et al. Risk of prostate cancer-specific mortality following biochemical recurrence after radical prostatectomy. *JAMA* 2005;294: 433–9.

Roach M 3rd, Hanks G, Thames H Jr et al. Defining biochemical failure following radiotherapy with or without hormonal therapy in men with clinically localized prostate cancer: recommendations of the RTOG-ASTRO Phoenix Consensus Conference. *Int J Radiat Oncol Biol Phys* 2006;65:965–74.

Sridharan S, Steigler A, Spry NA et al. Oligometastatic bone disease in prostate cancer patients treated on the TROG 03.04 RADAR trial. *Radiother Oncol* 2016;121:98–102.

Stephenson AJ, Scardino PT, Kattan MW et al. Predicting the outcome of salvage radiation therapy for recurrent prostate cancer after radical prostatectomy. *J Clin Oncol* 2007;25:2035–41.

Thompson IM, Tangen CM, Paradelo J et al. Adjuvant radiotherapy for pathological T3N0M0 prostate cancer significantly reduces risk of metastases and improves survival: long-term followup of a randomized clinical trial. *J Urol* 2009;181: 956–62.

Van der Kwast TH, Bolla M, Van Poppel H et al. Identification of patients with prostate cancer who benefit from immediate postoperative radiotherapy: EORTC 22911. *J Clin Oncol* 2007;25: 4178–86.

Although there is a trend towards earlier detection of prostate cancer, many men worldwide still present with widespread metastatic disease. In countries where prostate-specific antigen (PSA) testing is not widely used, about 30% of patients present with localized disease, 40% with locally advanced disease and the remaining 30% with metastases. In contrast to localized or locally advanced disease, metastatic prostate cancer is associated with high mortality – approximately 70% within 5 years. Androgen deprivation, which has become the mainstay of treatment, effectively reduces the intratumoral dihydrotestosterone (DHT) concentration by 70–80%, reducing stimulation of androgen receptors and increasing apoptosis of prostate cancer cells (Table 7.1). Androgen deprivation can be achieved by orchidectomy (surgical removal of the testes) or treatment with luteinizing hormone-releasing hormone (LHRH) analogs/antagonists; the value of adding an antiandrogen (maximal androgen blockade; see page 90) is still debated.

Some of the trials with important results for the treatment of metastatic prostate cancer are summarized at the end of this chapter (see Table 7.4).

## Orchidectomy

Bilateral orchidectomy or bilateral subcapsular orchidectomy is performed through a midline scrotal incision (Figure 7.1) under local, regional or light general anesthesia. The procedure is simple and is associated with little morbidity. The principal adverse events are local complications such as hematoma and wound infections, together with the usual effects of androgen deprivation such as loss of libido, erectile dysfunction and hot flashes (Table 7.2). Clinical responses (decreased bone pain and reduced PSA concentration) are obtained in more than 75% of patients. Because of the psychological/cosmetic impact of orchidectomy and its irreversibility, however, most patients and their partners prefer non-surgical treatment with LHRH analogs/antagonists.

TABLE 7.1

**Treatment options for metastatic prostate cancer**

- Androgen deprivation
  - Orchidectomy
  - LHRH analogs
  - LHRH antagonists
- Androgen deprivation and chemotherapy
- Maximal androgen blockade
- Intermittent androgen blockade
- Combination with docetaxel chemotherapy

LHRH, luteinizing hormone-releasing hormone.

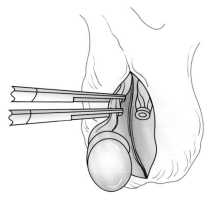

**Figure 7.1** Bilateral orchidectomy is generally performed via a midline scrotal incision.

TABLE 7.2

**Side effects of androgen-deprivation therapy**

- Hot flashes
- Decreased libido
- Lethargy
- Cognitive decline
- Mood changes
- Osteoporosis
- Weight gain
- Loss of muscle mass

## LHRH analogs

LHRH analogs, such as goserelin acetate, buserelin and leuprorelin (leuprolide acetate), are highly potent LHRH agonists (superagonists). Administration is followed by an initial transient increase in the secretion of luteinizing hormone (LH), and hence in testosterone, which lasts about 3 weeks, but this is followed by desensitization (downregulation), resulting in decreased secretion of LH and testosterone (Figure 7.2). These agents can be delivered via 1-, 3- or 6-monthly depot preparations, administered subcutaneously or intramuscularly. A potential side effect is tumor 'flare' resulting from the initial transient increase (140–170%) in testosterone, experienced by 8–32% of patients. This may result in increased bone

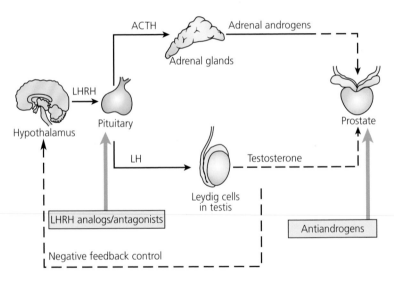

**Figure 7.2** Luteinizing hormone-releasing hormone (LHRH) analogs initially stimulate the release of luteinizing hormone (LH) and thus testosterone secretion ('flare'), but then desensitize the pituitary LHRH receptors, resulting in a fall in LH, and thus testosterone, levels. LHRH antagonists compete with naturally occurring LHRH to bind to the pituitary LHRH receptors, preventing the release of LH. This leads to a rapid suppression of testosterone release from the testes. Antiandrogens act peripherally to block testosterone action on androgen receptors. ACTH, adrenocorticotropic hormone.

pain or worsening symptoms of bladder outflow or ureteric obstruction; spinal metastases may also be stimulated to expand, increasing the risk of spinal cord compression. Tumor flare can be avoided by prior and concomitant administration of an antiandrogen during the first 4–6 weeks of LHRH analog treatment.

Comparative trials have shown that the response rates obtained with LHRH analogs are equivalent to those obtained after orchidectomy in terms of time to progression and OS. However, the reduction in testosterone may induce features of the metabolic syndrome (see page 126) and reduce bone mineral density (BMD; see page 125).

## LHRH antagonists

Pure LHRH (or gonadotropin-releasing hormone) antagonists block pituitary receptors and thereby inhibit LHRH release without causing the initial stimulation in LH and testosterone seen with the LHRH analogs; thus, they are not associated with a surge in testosterone (flare). The LHRH antagonist degarelix has shown positive clinical results in controlled clinical studies involving men with hormone-sensitive prostate cancer (Figure 7.3). A rapid reduction in testosterone without flare was achieved with this antagonist, compared with the significant flare associated with an LHRH analog. PSA decrease was rapid in both cases and was maintained in the long term.

LHRH antagonists are particularly beneficial for patients with bony metastases, spinal cord compression or bladder neck obstruction, for whom rapid tumor control without testosterone surge is important. An additional potential benefit could be in men receiving intermittent hormonal therapy, in whom the rapid return to normal LHRH receptor function following withdrawal of the drug results in an accompanying rapid return of testosterone. Recently, it has been suggested that LHRH antagonists carry a lower risk of cardiovascular side effects than the LHRH analogs, possibly because they maintain consistently low testosterone levels.

## Antiandrogens

Antiandrogens (taken in tablet form) do not alter the levels of circulating androgens. Instead, they inhibit the androgen receptor

89

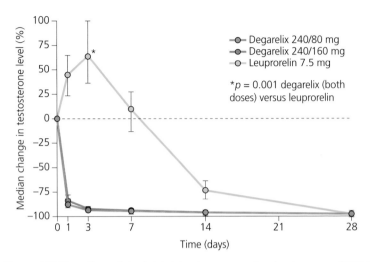

**Figure 7.3** The effect of the luteinizing hormone-releasing hormone (LHRH) antagonist degarelix on testosterone level. At a starting dose of 240 mg, followed by a monthly maintenance dose of either 80 mg or 160 mg, degarelix reduced serum testosterone level more rapidly than leuprorelin, 7.5 mg monthly. This phase III trial involved 610 men with prostate cancer (any stage). Reproduced with permission from Klotz et al. 2008.

where testosterone or DHT binds. They may be steroidal or non-steroidal.

- The steroidal antiandrogens (e.g. cyproterone acetate) also have a central testosterone-lowering effect and can be taken as monotherapy instead of castration, although they are not as effective.
- The non-steroidal antiandrogens inhibit the androgen receptor only and should not be taken as monotherapy for metastatic disease as the results are inferior to those achieved with LHRH analogs.

### Maximal androgen blockade

Although both orchidectomy and LHRH treatment produce dramatic initial responses in 70–80% of men, remission is not usually maintained in the long term. Androgen-independent cancer cell clones are selected out, and the mean time to tumor progression is less than 18 months and mean overall survival (OS) is 28–36 months. Persistent adrenal androgen secretion may contribute to this poor prognosis; there is evidence that adrenal androgens account for up to 15–20% of total androgen concentrations within the prostate. This has led to the concept of 'maximal androgen blockade', in which androgen deprivation by orchidectomy or LHRH treatment is accompanied by treatment with an antiandrogen to block the effects of adrenal androgens in the prostate.

Several trials have shown that maximal androgen blockade using an LHRH analog in combination with an antiandrogen improves survival compared with either LHRH analog treatment alone or orchidectomy. However, other trials have not shown significant improvements in tumor progression and survival, and a meta-analysis of all studies demonstrated little or no advantage with the combined therapy. This discrepancy may arise from steroidal and non-steroidal antiandrogens being evaluated together – a subgroup analysis of combination treatment with non-steroidal antiandrogens showed a small survival advantage of 2.9% for combination therapy compared with monotherapy.

In addition, maximal androgen blockade may offer a slight advantage over monotherapy in a subgroup of patients with good performance status (i.e. those who are generally well) and a relatively restricted metastatic burden. Such treatment should therefore be considered in younger and fitter patients who are more likely to die from the prostate cancer rather than from a comorbid condition. However, the relatively modest benefits need to be weighed against the increased costs and the small but significant incidence in side effects from the antiandrogens.

## The timing of hormonal therapy

The appropriate timing of hormonal therapy has been the subject of vigorous debate and the evidence now favors earlier therapy rather than waiting for symptoms. This evidence includes a re-analysis of the cooperative studies (USA) in which men receiving diethylstilbestrol (DES), 1 mg, had a survival advantage. The Medical Research Council (UK) study showed that men with locally advanced or metastatic

TABLE 7.3

**Prostate-cancer-related complications in men with locally advanced or metastatic disease randomized to immediate or delayed hormone therapy**

| | Immediate hormone therapy (n = 469) | Delayed hormone therapy (n = 465) |
|---|---|---|
| Pathological fracture | 11 | 21 |
| Cord compression | 9 | 23 |
| Ureteric obstruction | 33 | 55 |
| Development of extraskeletal metastases | 37 | 55 |

Adapted from the Medical Research Council Prostate Cancer Working Party Investigators Group, 1997.

disease treated with castration at diagnosis had better outcomes than those in whom therapy was deferred (Table 7.3), and a US trial reported by Messing et al. in 2006 found that delayed hormonal treatment in men with pelvic lymph node metastases was associated with a sevenfold increase in deaths from prostate cancer compared with those who had immediate androgen ablation therapy. A study that explored the timing of androgen deprivation therapy (ADT) in men who experienced a rising PSA after primary treatment of prostate cancer reported a 45% decrease in OS in those who delayed therapy (by ≥ 2 years) compared with those who had immediate treatment.

It is clear that early initiation of hormone therapy in men with locally advanced or metastatic disease improves survival and decreases complications. It should be borne in mind, however, that earlier treatment with hormonal therapy increases the risk of side effects such as osteoporosis.

## Intermittent hormonal therapy

It has been suggested that continuous androgen ablation therapy may, in fact, increase the rate of progression of prostate cancer to a castrate-resistant state (see Chapter 8), prompting the exploration of the use of intermittent hormonal therapy, which also has the potential advantage of decreasing the side effects of therapy. In this approach, hormone therapy is initially given for 6–9 months. If PSA levels become normalized, the LHRH analog/antagonist is temporarily discontinued. Hormone therapy is resumed when serum PSA returns to pretreatment levels in those with a PSA below 20 ng/mL at diagnosis, or when PSA exceeds 20 ng/mL in patients with an initial PSA above this. Such a regimen allows serum testosterone to return to normal, thereby stimulating atrophic cells and rendering them more sensitive to androgen ablation (Figure 7.4).

The use of a pure LHRH antagonist, which blocks the receptor without initial stimulation (see page 89), could be advantageous in this setting given the absence of flare and, potentially, a more rapid restoration of testosterone level after cessation of therapy.

In some studies of intermittent hormonal therapy, up to five treatment cycles were given before evidence of castrate resistance appeared; men spent approximately 50% of the time off therapy.

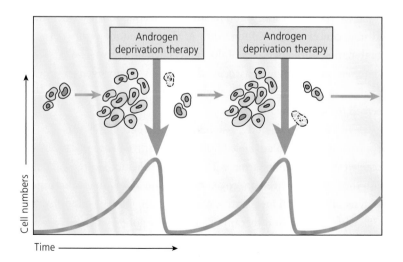

**Figure 7.4** Intermittent androgen ablation therapy allows serum testosterone to return periodically to normal, thereby stimulating atrophic cells and rendering them sensitive to subsequent androgen ablation.

Two randomized trials have compared intermittent versus continuous treatment in men with advanced prostate cancer. The first study, from Canada, included 1386 men with a rising PSA after failure of radiotherapy, who were randomized to continuous or intermittent hormone therapy. Survival was approximately 9 years, and was similar between the groups; however, the group receiving intermittent treatment had better quality of life in the areas of physical function, fatigue, hot flashes, libido and erectile function. The results from a US study of 1535 men with metastatic prostate cancer who were randomized to continuous or intermittent hormone treatment were statistically inconclusive, although there was a trend for longer survival in men receiving continuous treatment (5.8 years, vs 5.1 years in men receiving intermittent treatment). It appears that intermittent hormone therapy is safe and preferable in men with a rising PSA level, whereas men with confirmed metastatic disease may be better treated with continuous therapy.

Management of the adverse effects of ADT is described in Chapter 9.

## Androgen deprivation in combination with chemotherapy

In the CHAARTED study, 790 men with hormone-sensitive metastatic prostate cancer were randomized to ADT, either alone or in combination with six cycles of docetaxel chemotherapy. The combination therapy was associated with a 33% improvement in OS (median 58 vs 44 months). Men who had a high volume of metastases seemed to benefit the most.

In the STAMPEDE study, a significant difference in OS was reported in men with advanced hormone-sensitive prostate cancer who received ADT in combination with docetaxel chemotherapy compared with those who received androgen deprivation alone. In a subgroup analysis of men with metastatic prostate cancer, OS was improved by 27% with combination therapy. There is now good evidence that, at least in men with high-volume hormone-sensitive metastatic prostate cancer, giving early docetaxel chemotherapy in addition to androgen deprivation therapy improves survival.

## Spinal cord compression and pathological fractures

Sudden onset of low back pain and weakness in the lower limbs, with or without voiding difficulty, in a patient with metastatic prostate cancer is a urologic/neurosurgical emergency. Spinal cord compression due to pathological fracture or collapse of the lumbar vertebrae is the most common reason for these symptoms (Figure 7.5). The diagnosis may be confirmed by urgent spinal MRI. Early neurosurgical decompression is often advised, usually followed by external-beam radiotherapy (EBRT) and corticosteroids.

Pathological fractures caused by prostate cancer metastases may also occur elsewhere, such as in the femur or humerus. Fixation by an orthopedic specialist is often required and should usually be followed by EBRT and androgen ablation.

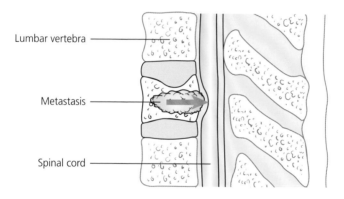

Lumbar vertebra

Metastasis

Spinal cord

**Figure 7.5** Spinal cord compression as a result of a spinal metastasis.

TABLE 7.4

**Important trials in the treatment of metastatic prostate cancer**

| Med/Comp | Trial | Use | Key outcomes |
|---|---|---|---|
| LHRH agonist/ Orchidectomy | Seidenfeld et al., 2000 | Metastatic prostate cancer | • Systematic review and meta-analysis of ten trials<br>• LHRH agonist demonstrated equivalent survival to orchidectomy (HR 1.12 [0.91–1.39]) |
| Maximal androgen blockade (MAB)/ Monotherapy androgen suppression | Prostate Cancer Trialists' Collaborative Group, 2000 | Metastatic prostate cancer | • Meta-analysis of 27 trials and 8275 men<br>• 2.9% survival increase for men treated with MAB (non-steroidal) vs monotherapy<br>• 2.8% survival decrease if MAB with cyproterone acetate used |
| Early hormonal therapy/Delayed hormonal therapy | MRC Prostate Cancer Working Party Investigators Group, 1997 | Locally advanced and metastatic prostate cancer | • Randomized trial of 938 men<br>• 257 men died from prostate cancer in the delayed treatment arm vs 203 in the early treatment arm ($p = 0.001$)<br>• The difference was largely seen in the men with stage C disease<br>• Complications from prostate cancer were almost halved in men receiving early treatment |
| Early hormonal therapy/Delayed hormonal therapy | Messing et al., 2006 | Men with pathologically involved lymph nodes after radical prostatectomy | • 98 men randomized to early vs delayed hormone therapy<br>• At 11.9 years' follow-up there was significant improvement in overall survival (HR 1.84 [1.01–3.35]); prostate-cancer-specific survival (HR 4.09 [1.76–9.49]) |

CONTINUED

TABLE 7.4 (CONTINUED)

## Important trials in the treatment of metastatic prostate cancer

| Med/Comp | Trial | Use | Key outcomes |
|---|---|---|---|
| Intermittent hormone therapy/ Continuous hormone therapy | Crook et al., 2012 | Men with rising PSA after radio-therapy | • 1386 men randomized to intermittent vs continuous hormone therapy<br>• Intermittent: significant quality-of-life benefits<br>• Median survival 8.8 vs 9.1 years for intermittent vs continuous (not significant) |
| Intermittent hormone therapy/ Continuous hormone therapy | Hussain et al., 2013 | Metastatic prostate cancer | • 1535 men randomized to intermittent vs continuous hormone therapy<br>• At median follow-up of 9.8 years, survival was 5.1 vs 5.8 years in the intermittent and continuous groups, respectively (HR 1.1 [0.99–1.23])<br>• Intermittent: significant improvements in mental function and erectile function |
| Combination with docetaxel/ Continuous hormone therapy | Sweeney et al., 2015 | Metastatic hormone-naïve prostate cancer | • Randomized trial of 790 men with metastatic hormone-naïve prostate cancer<br>• Addition of six cycles of chemotherapy to ADT improved survival by 39% |
| Combination with docetaxel/ Continuous hormone therapy | James et al., 2016 | Metastatic hormone-naïve prostate cancer | • Randomized trial of 2962 men with metastatic hormone-sensitive prostate cancer<br>• Men treated with six cycles of docetaxel in addition to standard of care (ADT) experienced 22% improvement in survival |

Seidenfeld J et al. *Ann Intern Med* 2000;132:566–77.
Prostate Cancer Trialists' Collaborative Group. *Lancet* 2000;355:1491–8.
The Medical Research Council Prostate Cancer Working Party Investigators Group. *Br J Urol* 1997;79:235–46.
Messing EM et al. *Lancet Oncol* 2006;7:472–9.
Crook JM et al. *N Engl J Med* 2012;367:895–903.
Hussain M et al. *N Engl J Med* 2013;368:1314–25.
Sweeny CJ et al. *New Engl J Med* 2015;373:737–46.
James N et al. *Lancet* 2016;387:1163–77.

ADT, androgen deprivation therapy; Comp, comparator; HR, hazard ratio; LHRH, luteinizing hormone-releasing hormone; Med, medication; MRC, Medical Research Council.

**Key points – management of metastatic prostate cancer**

- Treatment of metastatic prostate cancer is usually by androgen ablation.
- A luteinizing hormone-releasing hormone (LHRH) analog preceded and then accompanied by an antiandrogen is the most frequent treatment strategy.
- Treatment with a pure LHRH antagonist is another option, which avoids the need for an antiandrogen.
- Responses in terms of prostate-specific antigen (PSA) reduction and clinical improvement are seen in more than 80% of patients.
- Men with a high volume of metastases should be treated with a combination of androgen deprivation therapy and docetaxel chemotherapy.
- Eventually, androgen-insensitive cell clones develop and the PSA level begins to rise (castrate resistance).
- The side effects of medical castration include hot flashes, loss of libido and erectile dysfunction, and the reduced testosterone level may also be associated with features of the metabolic syndrome.

**Key references**

Also see Table 7.4.

Calais da Silva FE, Bono AV, Whelan P et al. Intermittent androgen deprivation for locally advanced and metastatic prostate cancer: results from a randomised phase 3 study of the South European Uroncological Group. *Eur Urol* 2009;55:1269–77.

Denis LD, Carneiro de Moura JL, Bono A et al. Goserelin acetate and flutamide versus bilateral orchidectomy: a phase III EORTC trial (30853). *Urology* 1993;42: 119–29.

Diamond E, Garcias Mdel C, Karir B, Tagawa ST. The evolving role of cytotoxic chemotherapy in the management of patients with metastatic prostate cancer. *Curr Treat Options Oncol* 2015;16:9.

Duchesne GM, Woo HH, Bassett JK et al. Timing of androgen-deprivation therapy in patients with prostate cancer with a rising PSA (TROG 03.06 and VCOG PR 01-03 [TOAD]): a randomised, multicentre, non-blinded, phase 3 trial. *Lancet Oncol* 2016;1:727–37.

Holmes-Walker DJ, Woo H, Gurney H et al. Maintaining bone health in patients with prostate cancer. *Med J Aust* 2006;184:176–9.

Klotz L, Boccon-Gibod L, Shore ND et al. The efficacy and safety of degarelix: a 12 month, comparative randomised, open-label, parallel-group phase III study in prostate cancer patients. *BJU Int* 2008;102:1531–8.

Langenhuijsen J, Schasfoort E, Heathcote P et al. Intermittent androgen suppression in patients with advanced prostate cancer: an update of the TULP survival data. *Eur Urol (suppl)* 2008;7:205 (abstr 538).

Messing EM, Manola J, Yao J et al. Immediate versus deferred androgen deprivation treatment in patients with node-positive prostate cancer after radical prostatectomy and pelvic lymphadenectomy. *Lancet Oncol.* 2006;7:472–9.

Mittan D, Lee S, Miller E et al. Bone loss following hypogonadism in men with prostate cancer treated with GnRH analogs. *J Clin Endocrinol Metab* 2002;87:3656–61.

Prostate Cancer Trialists' Collaborative Group. Maximum androgen blockade in advanced prostate cancer: an overview of 22 randomized trials with 3283 deaths in 5710 patients. *Lancet* 1995; 346:265–9.

Prostate Cancer Trialists' Collaborative Group. Maximum androgen blockade in advanced prostate cancer: an overview of the randomised trials. *Lancet* 2000;355:1491–8.

Sweeney CJ, Chen YH, Carducci M et al. Chemohormonal therapy in metastatic hormone-sensitive prostate cancer. *N Engl J Med* 2015; 373:737–46.

Tombal B, Miller K, Boccon-Gibod L et al. Additional analysis of the secondary end point of biochemical recurrence rate in a phase 3 trial (CS21) comparing degarelix 80 mg versus leuprolide in prostate cancer patients segmented by baseline characteristics. *Eur Urol* 2010;57:836–42.

Trachtenberg J, Gittleman M, Steidle C et al. A phase 3, multicenter, open label, randomized study of abarelix versus leuprolide plus daily antiandrogen in men with prostate cancer. *J Urol* 2002;167:1670–4.

# 8 Management of castrate-resistant prostate cancer

In most cases, advanced prostate cancers treated with any form of androgen-deprivation therapy (ADT) eventually begin to progress, a phenomenon known as 'castrate resistance'. An increase in prostate-specific antigen (PSA) level after initially successful androgen deprivation almost inevitably indicates impending clinical progression. Castrate-resistant prostate cancer (CRPC) has been characterized as disease that has progressed despite the persistence of castrate levels of androgens (< 1.73 nmol/L or 50 ng/dL), but remains hormone sensitive and is amenable to further hormonal manipulation. This state probably arises from either clonal selection of androgen-independent cell lines (Figure 8.1) or increased ligand-independent activation of androgen receptors.

Men with CRPC are a heterogeneous group, ranging from men with increasing PSA only and no demonstrable metastases to those who have many bone and/or visceral metastases (Figure 8.2), pain and poor functional status. Survival can range from only a few months to

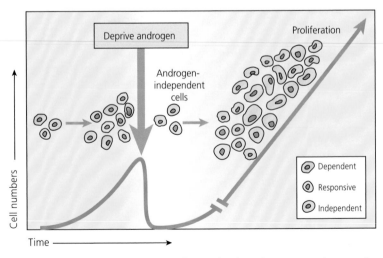

**Figure 8.1** Hormone escape results from selection of castrate-resistant cells.

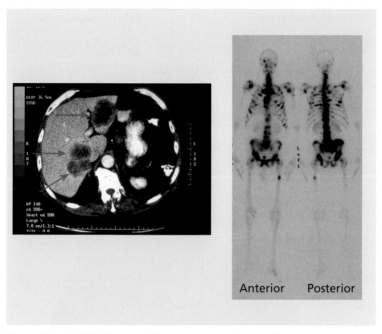

Anterior     Posterior

**Figure 8.2** Multiple bone and liver metastases (arrowed) in castrate-resistant prostate cancer.

4 years or more. Historically, therapy had little effect beyond modest palliation. More recently, however, several new treatment options have become available that not only improve quality of life and reduce pain but also increase survival (Figure 8.3). Some of the trials with important results for the treatment of CRPC are summarized in Table 8.1.

## Further hormonal manipulation

**Antiandrogens.** When the serum PSA level rises after a period of ADT alone, an initial step may be to add an antiandrogen to the treatment. This may transiently reduce PSA, but the PSA will usually start to rise again relatively soon. Withdrawal of the antiandrogen at this time produces a favorable PSA response in approximately 40% of men for 4–6 months. This phenomenon has been ascribed to a mutation affecting androgen receptors in malignant tissue which means that the antiandrogen acts as an agonist (stimulatory) rather than an

101

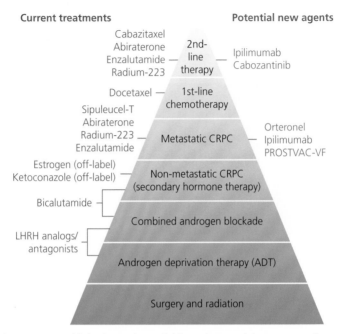

**Figure 8.3** Established, newly available and potential treatments for castrate-resistant prostate cancer (CRPC). LHRH, luteinizing hormone-releasing hormone. Adapted from Shore N et al. 2012.

antagonist (blocker), so when the antiandrogen is withdrawn the stimulation is reduced; a similar phenomenon occurs in breast cancer treated with antiestrogens. As long as the patient is asymptomatic, the addition and withdrawal of different antiandrogens can be continued for 2–3 cycles, as previous antiandrogen administration does not appear to diminish the response to different antiandrogens.

**Adrenal androgen synthesis inhibitors.** Antiandrogen withdrawal followed by inhibitors of adrenal androgen synthesis, such as aminoglutethimide or ketoconazole, has been shown to result in good reductions in PSA levels. However, adrenal androgen synthesis inhibitors are very toxic and not well tolerated, so this is not a usual treatment option.

TABLE 8.1

**Important trials in the treatment of castrate-resistant prostate cancer**

| Med/Comp | Trial | Use | Key outcomes |
|---|---|---|---|
| Docetaxel (chemotherapy), 3-weekly schedule/ Mitoxantrone plus prednisone | Tannock et al., 2004 (TAX–327); 1006 men randomized | First-line M1 CRPC | • Decreased disease progression and PSA response<br>• Increased pain improvement and quality of life<br>• Improved survival (18.9 vs 16.4 months; 24% relative reduction in death)<br>• Increased incidence of neutropenia, skin reactions and GI problems |
| Cabazitaxel (chemotherapy)/ Mitoxantrone | de Bono et al., 2010 (TROPIC); 755 men randomized | Second-line M1 CRPC | • Improved survival (15.1 vs 12.7 months), 30% RR for death<br>• Neutropenia and diarrhea were the most common side effects |
| Mitoxantrone plus prednisone (chemotherapy)/ Prednisone | Tannock et al., 1996; 161 men randomized | First-line M1 CRPC | • No difference in survival observed<br>• Significant improvement in palliative response and quality of life |
| Abiraterone plus prednisone (AR targeted)/ Placebo plus prednisone | Ryan et al., 2013; 1088 men randomized | M1 CRPC before chemo-therapy | • Improved PFS (16.5 vs 8.3 months), RR for death 47%<br>• Improved OS (median not reached vs 27.2 months), RR for death 25%<br>• Delayed the initiation of chemotherapy |

CONTINUED

103

TABLE 8.1 (CONTINUED)

**Important trials in the treatment of castrate-resistant prostate cancer**

| Med/Comp | Trial | Use | Key outcomes |
|---|---|---|---|
| Abiraterone plus prednisone (AR targeted)/ Placebo plus prednisone | de Bono et al., 2011; 1195 men randomized 2:1 | Following docetaxel chemotherapy in M1 CRPC | • Increased survival (14.8 vs 10.9 months), RR for death 35% <br> • Mineralocorticoid-related AEs, including fluid retention, hypertension and hypokalemia |
| Enzalutamide (AR targeted)/ Placebo | Scher et al., 2012 (AFFIRM); 1199 men randomized | Following docetaxel chemotherapy in M1 CRPC | • Improved OS (18.4 vs 13.6 months), RR for death 37% <br> • Improvements in PSA response, soft tissue response, quality of life and time to first SRE <br> • Side effects of fatigue, diarrhea, hot flashes and, rarely, seizures |
| Enzalutamide (AR targeted)/ Placebo | Kimura et al., 2016 (PREVAIL); 1717 men randomized | M1 CRPC before chemotherapy | • Improved radiographic PFS (65% vs 14%) <br> • Survival improved by 29% in those randomized to enzalutamide |
| Sipuleucel-T (immuno-therapy)/ Placebo | Kantoff et al., 2010; 512 men randomized | M1 CRPC | • Improved survival (25.8 vs 21.7 months), RR for death 22% <br> • Treatment side effects were minimal |

CONTINUED

TABLE 8.1 (CONTINUED)

## Important trials in the treatment of castrate-resistant prostate cancer

| Med/Comp | Trial | Use | Key outcomes |
|---|---|---|---|
| Radium-223 (targeted alpha therapy)/Placebo | Parker et al., 2013 (ALSYMPCA); 921 men randomized | M1 CRPC | • Improved OS (14.9 vs 11.3 months), HR 0.70, RR for death 30%<br><br>• Associated with low myelosuppression rates and fewer AEs |
| Zoledronic acid (bisphosphonate), 4 mg or 8 mg/ Placebo | Saad et al., 2002; 643 men randomized 1:1:1 | M1 CRPC | • Median time to first SRE event increased with 4 mg vs 8 mg vs placebo (not reached vs 363 days vs 321 days)<br><br>• Pain and analgesic scores higher in placebo group |
| Denosumab (monoclonal antibody)/ Zoledronic acid | Fizazi et al., 2011; 1904 men randomized | M1 CRPC | • Increased median time to first SRE (20.7 vs 17.1 months), HR 0.82<br><br>• AEs equivalent in both arms |

Tannock IF et al. *N Engl J Med* 2004;351:1502–12.
de Bono JS et al. *Lancet* 2010;376:1147–54.
Tannock IF et al. *J Clin Oncol* 1996;14:1756–64.
Ryan CJ et al. *N Engl J Med* 2013;368:138–48.
de Bono JS et al. *N Engl J Med* 2011;364:1995–2005.
Scher HI et al. *N Engl J Med* 2012;367:1187–97.
Kimura G *Int J Urol* 2016;23:395–403.
Kantoff PW et al. *N Engl J Med* 2010;363:411–22.
Parker C et al. *N Engl J Med* 2013;369:213–23.
Saad F et al. *J Natl Cancer Inst* 2002;94:1458–68.
Fizazi K et al. *Lancet* 2011;377:813–22.

AE, adverse event; AR, androgen receptor; Comp, comparator; CRPC, castrate-resistant prostate cancer; GI, gastrointestinal; HR, hazard ratio; Med, medication; OS, overall survival; PFS, progression-free survival; PSA, prostate-specific antigen; RR, relative risk; SRE, skeletal-related event.

**Estrogen** treatment may benefit some men with CRPC. It appears to have two effects:

- inhibition of pituitary gonadotropin secretion
- direct cytotoxic effect on the tumor.

The synthetic estrogen diethylstilbestrol (DES) has been used in prostate cancer but its use in first-line therapy is limited by side effects such as gynecomastia, deep-vein thrombosis and other cardiovascular complications. A combination of DES with acetylsalicylic acid (ASA; aspirin) or warfarin may reduce the thrombotic and cardiovascular toxicity, which can be particularly hazardous in men of this age, but patients should be alerted to the risks.

### Non-metastatic (M0) castrate-resistant prostate cancer

Men who start ADT before any metastases are found, such as for a rising PSA after radiotherapy, may become castrate resistant without any evidence of distant metastases (M0 CRPC). These men can present a difficult management dilemma, because the rising PSA can cause significant psychological distress, even though they are asymptomatic.

Traditionally, treatment has been either further hormonal manipulation, as described above, or treatment within a clinical trial. Once these fail, however, an observational approach is taken until the patient develops demonstrable metastases (M1 CRPC) for which further treatments are available (see below).

Although a number of therapies, such as the endothelin antagonists atrasentan and zibotentan, have been trialed, none has been effective in delaying the progression of M0 CRPC to M1 CRPC. A plethora of new drugs are being evaluated and, with time, it is possible that one or more may be effective for this disease stage.

### Metastatic (M1) castrate-resistant prostate cancer

**Abiraterone** is approved as first-line treatment for metastatic CRPC. It is a specific inhibitor of cytochrome P450 17-hydroxylase/17,20-lyase (CYP17), a key enzyme in androgen synthesis (Figure 8.4). Abiraterone is effective in CRPC because, despite castrate levels of circulating androgens from luteinizing hormone-releasing hormone

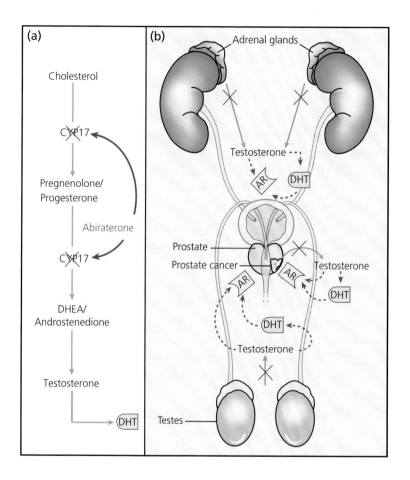

**Figure 8.4** (a) Androgen biosynthesis. By inhibiting the action of cytochrome P450 17-hydroxylase/17,20-lyase (CYP17) – a key enzyme in the biosynthesis of androgens from cholesterol – abiraterone interferes with the production of dehydroepiandrosterone (DHEA) and androstenedione, precursors of testosterone and dihydrotestosterone (DHT). (b) While castration leads to decreased production of testosterone and DHT by the testes, the adrenal glands and prostate cancer tissue continue to produce these androgens, leading to activation of androgen receptors (ARs) and continued growth of prostate cancer. Abiraterone blocks the production of testosterone and DHT via the pathway shown in (a) at all three of these sites, thus providing an alternative treatment for patients with castrate-resistant disease.

(LHRH) agonist/antagonist therapy, CRPC cells synthesize their own androgens from cholesterol, which then perpetuate androgen receptor signaling.

In a randomized trial involving 1088 men with asymptomatic or mildly symptomatic metastatic CRPC who had not received previous chemotherapy, abiraterone plus prednisone improved radiographic progression-free survival and OS compared with prednisone alone; it also delayed PSA progression and increased the times to opiate use and initiation of cytotoxic chemotherapy (see Table 8.1). The incidence of grade 3/4 mineralocorticoid-related adverse events and liver-function abnormalities was higher in the group receiving abiraterone, but no unique toxic events occurred.

**Enzalutamide** is an androgen-receptor-signaling inhibitor, approved for the treatment of metastatic CRPC either prior to chemotherapy or after previous docetaxel treatment. It inhibits nuclear translocation of the androgen receptor, DNA binding and coactivator recruitment (Figure 8.5), and has a greater affinity for the receptor than non-steroidal antiandrogens; it does not have any agonist activity (see Table 8.1).

In the PREVAIL trial in men with metastatic CRPC who had not had prior chemotherapy, oral enzalutamide, 160 mg/day, was associated with a 29% improvement in survival compared with placebo. Enzalutamide was associated with fatigue, diarrhea and hot flashes.

**Docetaxel**, a member of the taxoid family, induces apoptosis through microtubule stabilization; it has been established as first-line therapy for M1 CRPC for many years. A randomized trial (TAX–327) in men with CRPC found that a 3-week schedule of docetaxel was superior to mitoxantrone plus prednisone in terms of disease progression and OS (see Table 8.1). The incidence of neutropenia, skin reactions and gastrointestinal problems was higher with docetaxel than with mitoxantrone plus prednisone. These are the most common side effects with docetaxel but in general the chemotherapeutic agent is well tolerated.

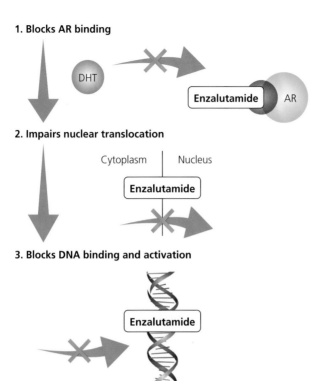

**1. Blocks AR binding**

DHT

Enzalutamide | AR

**2. Impairs nuclear translocation**

Cytoplasm | Nucleus

Enzalutamide

**3. Blocks DNA binding and activation**

Enzalutamide

**Figure 8.5** Mechanism of action of enzalutamide, which inhibits androgen receptor (AR) signaling in three ways. Based on Tran C et al. *Science* 2009; 324:787–90; and Watson PA et al. *Proc Natl Acad Sci USA*; 2010:107: 16759–65. DHT, dihydrotestosterone.

**Radium-223** delivers targeted alpha therapy to bones. It is approved for the treatment of CRPC in men with symptomatic bone metastases and no known visceral metastatic disease. As alpha particles have limited penetration, radium-223 delivers highly localized therapy, killing tumor cells but with minimal damage to surrounding tissue. The phase III ALSYMPCA study compared radium-223 with best supportive care (BSC) versus placebo with BSC in men with CRPC and bone metastases who had failed on or were unsuitable for docetaxel treatment. OS was improved with radium-223 (see Table 8.1); side effects included increased low-grade nausea, diarrhea and occasional neutropenia.

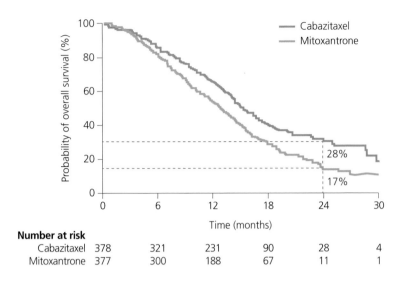

**Number at risk**

| | | | | | | |
|---|---|---|---|---|---|---|
| Cabazitaxel | 378 | 321 | 231 | 90 | 28 | 4 |
| Mitoxantrone | 377 | 300 | 188 | 67 | 11 | 1 |

**Figure 8.6** Overall survival in the TROPIC trial. At 2 years, 28% of patients in the cabazitaxel group were alive, compared with 17% in the mitoxantrone group. From de Bono JS et al. *Lancet* 2010;376:1147–54, reproduced with permission from Elsevier.

**Second-line therapy.** Treatment options when prostate cancer progresses after docetaxel chemotherapy include further chemotherapy, one of the new hormonal modulation agents or targeted alpha therapy.

*Cabazitaxel.* This taxane chemotherapy was developed to overcome the resistance that can develop as a result of docetaxel treatment. In the TROPIC study, men with CRPC that had progressed after docetaxel treatment were randomized to cabazitaxel or mitoxantrone. Those who received cabazitaxel demonstrated a 30% improvement in survival compared with those receiving mitoxantrone (15.1 versus 12.7 months; Figure 8.6 and see Table 8.1). Side effects were similar to those seen with docetaxel.

*Mitoxantrone and prednisone* was the first chemotherapy combination to be tested in a randomized trial in advanced prostate cancer. The combination was very well tolerated and more than doubled the time of palliation response compared with prednisone alone. It also improved the quality of life of men with CRPC. It has now been replaced by docetaxel as first-line chemotherapy and by cabazitaxel as second-line chemotherapy, which have better efficacy; however, the combination still has a place in second-line therapy when resistance to docetaxel has developed and cabazitaxel is not an option.

*Abiraterone.* In a study in men with metastatic CRPC for whom docetaxel chemotherapy had failed, abiraterone plus prednisone resulted in a 35% improvement in survival compared with prednisone alone (see Table 8.1). Mineralocorticoid-related adverse events, including fluid retention, hypertension and hypokalemia, were more frequent in the abiraterone group, highlighting the continuing dependency of CRPC on androgen-receptor signaling even after it has become castrate resistant (see Table 8.1).

*Enzalutamide.* In the AFFIRM trial, oral enzalutamide, 160 mg/day, improved survival in men with metastatic CRPC after failure of docetaxel chemotherapy (see Table 8.1). However, rates of fatigue, diarrhea and hot flashes were higher in the enzalutamide group. Enzalutamide is often used after failure of docetaxel chemotherapy, if not used prior to it.

*Radium-223* delivers targeted alpha therapy to bones, delaying symptomatic skeletal and skeletal-related events. It has also been shown to improve OS (see page 109).

## Immunotherapy

Therapies that modulate the immune system are showing considerable promise in trials of CRPC. These therapies take time to mediate an effect and are therefore best used in men with minimal or no symptoms.

**Sipuleucel-T** is an autologous cellular immunotherapy. In a phase III trial of men with CRPC not previously treated with docetaxel, treatment with sipuleucel-T resulted in a 22% relative reduction in the risk of death compared with placebo, with minimal side effects (see Table 8.1). This is the first immunotherapy to demonstrate a survival advantage in prostate cancer; however, treatment is complicated and requires a specialized laboratory, which makes it extremely expensive to administer.

**Ipilimumab.** Cytotoxic T-lymphocyte antigen-4 (CTLA-4), which is a negative regulator of T-cell activation, has emerged as a target for cancer immunotherapy. Ipilimumab is a fully human monoclonal antibody that specifically blocks the binding of CTLA-4 to its ligands, thereby augmenting T-cell activation and proliferation and resulting in tumor regression. Significant tumor responses with ipilimumab were seen in a phase II trial in men with metastatic CRPC. This immunotherapy is currently in phase III trials.

**PD-1/PD-L1 blockade.** Monoclonal antibodies directed against PD-1 (programmed cell death protein-1) or PD-L1 (programmed death ligand 1), such as nivolumab, pembrolizumab and atezolizumab, can reinforce anti-tumor immune response by stimulating the activity of effector T cells against cancer cells and the tumor micro-environment. Various PD-1/PD-L1 inhibitors are currently in phase II trials.

It is likely that a single immune therapy may not have sufficient activity against CRPC, and that combinations of CTLA-4 and PD-1/PD-L1 blockade will be required.

**PROSTVAC-VF** is a prostate cancer vaccine regimen, consisting of a recombinant vaccinia vector as a primary vaccination, followed by multiple booster vaccinations, employing a recombinant fowlpox vector. These vaccines stimulate an antigen-presenting cell-mediated immune response to PSA-expressing tumor cells. In a small randomized study of men with metastatic CRPC, those treated with PROSTVAC-VF had better OS than the placebo group (25.1 versus 16.6 months). These results are promising but need confirmation in larger randomized trials.

## Management of bone metastases

Bone pain is one of the most intractable problems associated with CRPC, and conventional analgesics do not always provide relief.

**Palliative radiotherapy.** Hormone-naïve disease is initially managed with ADT. However, some men do not get full resolution of pain, or may have painful bone metastases in the setting of CRPC.

*Focal external-beam radiotherapy* is a well-established treatment, providing rapid improvement in pain in up to 80% of men. Treatment can be given as either a single fraction or as multiple fractions over 2–3 weeks. This type of irradiation is associated with very few side effects.

*Wide-field radiation* may also be useful in patients with intractable diffuse pain. It can delay the progression of existing disease as well as slow the occurrence of new disease, but is associated with side effects such as pneumonitis, cataracts, nausea, vomiting and diarrhea in approximately 35% of patients, and severe, sometimes irreversible, hematological effects in 9%.

*Systemic radionuclide therapy* is a means of targeting multiple painful bone metastases by intravenous administration of a radionuclide (such as samarium-153) complexed to bone-avid molecules such as ethylenediamine tetra (methylene phosphonic acid) (EDTMP), or radionuclides that have a natural affinity for metabolically active bone, such as strontium-89. After administration of samarium-153, 65–80% of patients report relief from pain and symptoms within 1 week. The average duration of response is 2–3 months. The major toxicity is myelosuppression, which can last a number of months; white blood cell count and platelet levels should therefore be monitored before and after therapy.

*CyberKnife-targeted radiotherapy* is becoming increasingly popular for the targeted treatment of metastases that are solitary or low in numbers (i.e. oligometastases; see page 70).

**Bisphosphonates** suppress bone resorption and demineralization, providing symptomatic benefit in some patients. A study involving over 600 men with CRPC demonstrated a significant reduction in the number of patients with bone-related events among those receiving zoledronic acid (zoledronate), given as an intravenous infusion every 3 weeks, compared with placebo. Zoledronic acid also significantly delayed the onset of first skeletal-related event (see Table 8.1); however, the number needed to treat (NNT) to save one death is 10.

Side effects with bisphosphonates include renal deterioration and, rarely, osteonecrosis of the jaw.

**Denosumab** is a human monoclonal antibody directed against RANKL (receptor activator of nuclear factor κB ligand); it inhibits osteoclast function and bone turnover. A randomized trial involving 1904 men with CRPC supported denosumab as the optimal medication to reduce bone-related events in men with CRPC (see Table 8.1).

## Palliative care

Despite improving therapies, most patients with CRPC eventually die as a result of the cancer, often within 12–24 months. Treatment with high-dose steroids can sometimes provide useful palliation. The palliative care of these patients requires a supportive and caring team approach involving the family physician, the urologist, an experienced palliative care team and, of course, the patient's close relatives and friends.

## Treatment algorithm

A suggested algorithm for the treatment of CRPC is presented in Figure 8.7.

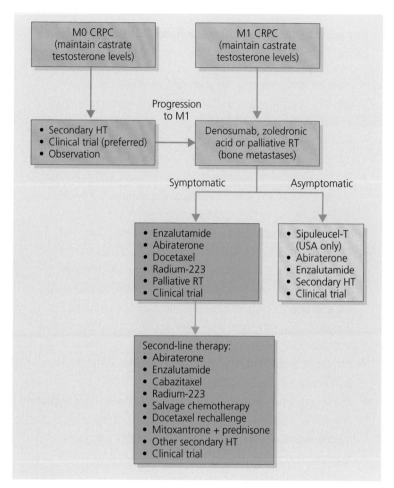

**Figure 8.7** Suggested treatment algorithm for men with castrate-resistant prostate cancer (CRPC). Adapted from Shore et al. *BJU Int* 2012;109(suppl):22–32. HT, hormone therapy; RT, radiotherapy.

**Key points – management of castrate-resistant prostate cancer**

- After an initial response to androgen ablation, the serum prostate-specific antigen (PSA) value starts to rise as a result of androgen-insensitive cell clones.
- As an initial step, withdraw any antiandrogen, then consider trying another antiandrogen.
- The mainstay of management for metastatic CRPC is docetaxel chemotherapy. The CYP17 inhibitor abiraterone is now also licensed for use before chemotherapy, and trials of other antiandrogens prior to chemotherapy are under way.
- When docetaxel chemotherapy has failed, second-line therapies such as cabazitaxel chemotherapy, abiraterone (a selective inhibitor of androgen biosynthesis), enzalutamide (an androgen-receptor-signaling inhibitor) and radium-223 (targeted alpha therapy) have been shown to improve survival and quality of life.
- Immunotherapy for CRPC may be best implemented before significant symptoms appear.
- The monoclonal antibody denosumab and the bisphosphonate zoledronic acid have been reported to significantly delay bone-related events in men with metastatic prostate cancer.
- External-beam radiotherapy may provide useful control of pain from bone metastases.

## Key references

Also see Table 8.1.

Fizazi K, Scher HI, Molina A et al. Abiraterone acetate for treatment of metastatic castration-resistant prostate cancer: final overall survival analysis of the COU-AA–301 randomised, double-blind, placebo-controlled phase 3 study. *Lancet Oncol* 2012;13:983–92.

Kantoff PW, Schuetz TJ, Blumenstein BA et al. Overall survival analysis of a phase II randomized controlled trial of a Poxviral-based PSA-targeted immunotherapy in metastatic castration-resistant prostate cancer. *J Clin Oncol* 2010;28:1099–105.

Lewington VJ, McEwan AJ, Ackery DM et al. A prospective, randomised double-blind crossover study to examine the efficacy of strontium-89 in pain palliation in patients with advanced prostate cancer metastatic to bone. *Eur J Cancer* 1991;27: 954–8.

Loriot Y, Miller K, Sternberg CN et al. Effect of enzalutamide on health-related quality of life, pain, and skeletal-related events in asymptomatic and minimally symptomatic, chemotherapy-naive patients with metastatic castration-resistant prostate cancer (PREVAIL): results from a randomised, phase 3 trial. *Lancet Oncol* 2015;16:509–21.

National Institute for Health and Care Excellence. Abiraterone for castration-resistant metastatic prostate cancer previously treated with a docetaxel-containing regimen. NICE Technology Appraisal No. 259. June 2012. http://guidance.nice. org.uk/TA259, last accessed 07 March 2017.

Parker C, Nilsson S, Heinrich D et al., for the ALSYMPCA Investigators. Alpha emitter radium-223 and survival in metastatic prostate cancer. *N Engl J Med* 2013;369:213–23.

Scher HI, Fizazi K, Saad F et al. Increased survival with enzalutamide in prostate cancer after chemotherapy. *N Engl J Med* 2012;367:1187–97.

Scher HI, Kelly WK. Flutamide withdrawal syndrome: its impact on clinical trials in hormone-refractory prostate cancer. *J Clin Oncol* 1993;11:1566–72.

Shore N, Mason M, de Reijke TM. New developments in castrate-resistant prostate cancer. *BJU Int* 2012;109(Suppl6):22–32.

Slovin SF, Higano CS, Hamid O et al. Ipilimumab alone or in combination with radiotherapy in metastatic castration-resistant prostate cancer: results from an open-label, multicenter phase I/II study. *Ann Oncol* 2013;24:1813–21.

Smith MR, Egerdie B, Hernandez Toriz N et al. Denosumab in men receiving androgen-deprivation therapy for prostate cancer. *N Engl J Med* 2009;361:745–55.

As more and more men with prostate cancer survive for longer and longer, 'survivorship' issues are becoming increasingly important. Primary care practitioners and allied healthcare professionals have an important role here: good management of treatment effects and complications can unquestionably improve the quality of life of affected men and should be incorporated into the routine care of all prostate cancer survivors. Remember, survivorship years can be some of the best years that patients have.

With this in mind, survivorship is not only about treating the tumor, but also about supporting the whole individual, as well as his immediate family, throughout the entire cancer journey. Psychological issues as well as medical matters need to be managed, including anxiety related to the cancer and its cure, depression, and fear of recurrence after treatment. In this respect, those who care for men with prostate cancer can learn a great deal from the teams and charities that treat and support those with breast cancer.

Other healthcare professionals, particularly urology nurse specialists, have a crucial role in encouraging prostate cancer survivors to share their concerns with loved ones, treatment teams, mental health professionals and prostate cancer support groups, as well as fellow survivors. Nurses also have a key role in referral of patients to the most appropriate advisory and support services.

## Sexual function
A diagnosis of prostate cancer alone may be enough to disrupt sexual activity which, in the age group usually affected, may already be waning.

**Erectile dysfunction.** Treatment of localized prostate cancer often results in sexual dysfunction. Erectile dysfunction is the most common complaint and can occur after all treatments. Improvements in techniques for radical prostatectomy and nerve sparing, such as the use of robotic assistance, have resulted in significant improvements in this area; however, erectile dysfunction can occur following even the most expert surgery. Unfortunately, it is also sometimes necessary to resect the cavernous nerves in order to avoid positive surgical margins, which can obviously have detrimental effects on erectile function.

Limited success has been reported with the replacement of resected nerves with sural nerve grafts after surgery in terms of erectile function (Figure 9.1). Newer synthetic products are in development however.

Intracorporeal fibrosis results from the release of transforming growth factor α (TGFα) in response to anoxia; thus, therapies that bring oxygenated arterial blood into the corpora and induce erection may inhibit the release of TGFα and help maintain smooth muscle function. Early administration of pharmaceutical treatments for erectile dysfunction soon after surgery has been shown to improve the time and quality of subsequent erections. Montorsi et al. have shown in a randomized trial that early intracavernosal injection of alprostadil (prostaglandin E$_1$), once or twice a week, results in early recovery of spontaneous erections after nerve-sparing radical prostatectomy. Early administration of phosphodiesterase type 5 (PDE5) inhibitors, such as tadalafil, 5 mg daily, has also been shown to improve the time and quality of spontaneous erections after bilateral nerve-sparing surgery.

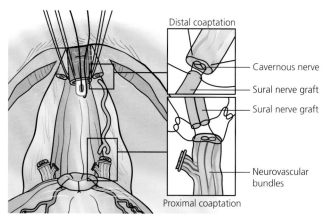

**Figure 9.1** Sural nerve graft interposition to restore erectile function following prostatectomy.

Patients refractory to intracavernosal and oral PDE5 inhibitor treatment have the option of using a vacuum constriction device to obtain erections, or surgery to insert an inflatable penile prosthesis (Figure 9.2).

External-beam radiotherapy (EBRT) and brachytherapy are both associated with an incidence of delayed-onset erectile dysfunction of 30% or more, and cryotherapy often results in erectile dysfunction because the neurovascular bundles are included in the freezing zone. Similarly, high-intensity focused ultrasonography (HIFU) can result in impaired erectile function if the neurovascular bundles are in the treated area. Treatment is along the same lines as that for erectile dysfunction following prostatectomy (see also *Fast Facts: Erectile Dysfunction*).

**Ejaculatory problems.** Men who undergo radical prostatectomy or transurethral resection of the prostate (TURP) for localized prostate cancer may also experience ejaculatory problems, although the sensation of orgasm is usually preserved. In the case of TURP, semen is still produced but passes retrogradely into the bladder. After radical prostatectomy, in which the entire prostate and seminal vesicles are removed, semen is not produced but most patients are still able to

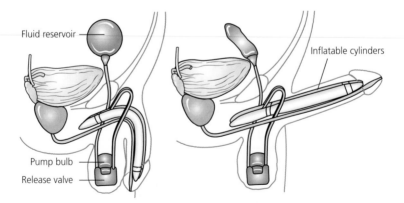

**Figure 9.2** An inflatable penile prosthesis. Squeezing the pump transfers fluid from the reservoir into the cylinders, causing an erection. Pushing the release valve drains the fluid back to the abdominal reservoir.

achieve orgasm. Patients must be informed about these consequences before surgery. Drugs such as the $\alpha_1$-blocker tamsulosin, used to treat bladder outflow obstruction, may also cause loss of, or reduced, ejaculation, but this is reversible on cessation of treatment.

**Loss of libido** is a common complaint in patients with prostate cancer. It may result from the disease itself causing debilitation or depression but, more commonly, it is a side effect of hormone ablation therapy. Bilateral orchidectomy or therapy with luteinizing hormone-releasing hormone (LHRH) analogs/antagonists is almost invariably associated with loss of libido, as well as erectile dysfunction. Therapy with an antiandrogen can effectively deprive prostate cancer cells of androgen stimulation without such a profound effect on libido or erectile function.

**Preservation of sexual function.** If this is an important factor in terms of the quality of life, treatment with an antiandrogen as monotherapy may well be considered as an alternative to bilateral orchidectomy or an LHRH analog.

**Counseling.** Men with prostate cancer, and their partners, should be counseled not only about probable outcomes, but also about the likely effect of the disease and its therapy on sexual activity. An open and informed approach to this important aspect of prostate cancer will do much to counter the anxiety and loss of self-esteem that often accompany the diagnosis of this prevalent malignancy, and to restore effective sexual function after treatment and thereby maintain an important aspect of quality of life.

## Urinary and bowel symptoms
**Incontinence following radical prostatectomy.** Radical prostatectomy involves removal of the prostate gland and some of the bladder neck, resulting in loss of the contribution of the bladder neck and prostatic smooth muscle to continence. Operative injury to the remaining rhabdosphincter or its nerve supply is probably the most common factor in post-prostatectomy incontinence. Other factors that may

contribute are bladder overactivity, which may have existed before surgery or developed after, and a poorly compliant bladder.

Some degree of immediate stress incontinence is expected following removal of the urethral catheter after surgery, but urinary control should improve gradually. The following factors contribute to the early recovery of continence:

- younger age of the patient
- an experienced surgeon
- bilateral nerve-sparing surgery
- absence of anastomotic stricture
- performing pelvic floor exercises before and after surgery.

Treatment is initially conservative, involving regulation of fluid intake, and pelvic floor exercises. Bladder overactivity can be treated with anticholinergic medication. If this fails, options include injection of a peri-urethral bulking agent, which has approximately 40% success in the short term, or insertion of a bulbo-urethral sling or artificial urinary sphincter (see *Fast Facts: Bladder Disorders*).

**Urinary and bowel symptoms from radiotherapy.** Irritative symptoms of urinary urgency and frequency are very common during the delivery of radiotherapy, and are considerably worse with high-dose-rate brachytherapy and seed brachytherapy than with EBRT; these symptoms tend to settle with time, however.

Later urinary symptoms include irritative symptoms such as urgency and frequency, pain and even incontinence and can be due to instability, poor compliance, urethral stricture, overflow incontinence, bladder ulcer or a combination of these. Brachytherapy in particular may result in persistent bladder outflow obstruction.

Rectal symptoms may also be troublesome after radiotherapy, and diarrhea, tenesmus and rectal bleeding may all occur. These tend to resolve over time but patients should be made aware that EBRT is associated with an increased risk of colorectal cancer. Persistent rectal bleeding should be investigated by colonoscopy.

Treatment is also initially conservative, and involves changes to lifestyle, identification of the cause and individualized treatment.

## Adverse effects of hormonal therapy

Prospective clinical trials of androgen deprivation therapy (ADT) in men with prostate cancer have highlighted multiple risk factors for bone health and cardiovascular disease, including increases in serum cholesterol and triglycerides, insulin resistance, body mass index and fat body mass, and decrease in lean body mass (Table 9.1).

**Hot flashes,** where a rise in the temperature of the face and trunk is accompanied by cutaneous vasodilatation – affecting mainly the face, throat and extremities – and sweating, are common in men using ADT. ADT-related hormone changes result in the release of catecholamines, notably norepinephrine, from the hypothalamus, which interferes with thermoregulation controlled by the upper hypothalamus.

Men should be counseled that hot flashes may continue despite efforts to overcome them, and advised to take steps to minimize the discomfort (e.g. wearing lighter clothing). Some hormonal treatments, such as the $\alpha_2$ receptor antagonist clonidine, may help, but all can have side effects that may outweigh the benefits. Progestins such as megestrol acetate seem to have the best side-effect profile. Other agents such as selective serotonin-reuptake inhibitors may also

TABLE 9.1

**Potential effects of androgen deprivation therapy**

| Metabolic effects | Physical changes |
|---|---|
| • Hyperlipidemia | • Increased fat mass |
| • Insulin resistance and diabetes | • Decreased muscle mass |
| • Osteoporosis | • Loss of body hair |
| • Increased risk of fracture | • Gynecomastia |
| • Anemia | • Hot flashes |
| **Mental changes** | **Sexual effects** |
| • Decreased cognition | • Decreased libido |
| • Emotional changes | • Erectile dysfunction |

be acceptable. There is currently little evidence to support the use of complementary therapies.

**Fatigue** resulting from hormone therapy is complex and overlaps with other side effects such as depression and pain. It can have a considerable impact on a man's quality of life as it may affect normal functioning and sleep.

Exercise and dietary advice constitute the first-line approach. Research has shown that following a regular exercise program can help overcome the weakness and muscle wasting that may develop with ADT, and can reduce the frequency and severity of fatigue. Often, the involvement of a dietitian and exercise physiologist can be beneficial. There is a suggestion that intermittent ADT may be associated with less fatigue than continuous ADT but this is not currently supported by strong trial evidence.

**Anemia** tends to be worse with maximum androgen blockade with combined LHRH agonist–antiandrogen than with either agent as monotherapy. Hemoglobin levels rise slowly after treatment has ended. Newly diagnosed men should have a blood count before starting ADT to check for pretreatment anemia and deficiencies in vitamin $B_{12}$, folate or iron, and hemoglobin levels should be monitored throughout ADT. Transfusions are recommended if hemoglobin is below 10 g/dL in symptomatic men, and in asymptomatic men with comorbidities such as congestive heart failure or cerebral vascular disease.

**Breast symptoms.** Men may experience gynecomastia and mastalgia (swollen and painful breasts) while using some forms of ADT. The likelihood varies with treatment; the risk is highest in men taking antiandrogens or estrogens.

In England and Wales, the National Institute for Health and Care Excellence (NICE) recommends prophylactic radiotherapy to both breast buds within the first month of long-term treatment with the antiandrogen bicalutamide (150 mg monotherapy for more than 6 months). While this makes sense as a palliative measure for men with advanced disease, for men with locally advanced disease, the advantages and disadvantages of prophylactic radiotherapy need careful consideration as there is a risk of a second malignancy, albeit theoretical in the absence of long-term data.

There is some evidence to support the use of tamoxifen prior to bicalutamide to reduce the development of breast symptoms. Surgical options include adenomammectomy with periareolar incision, and incision and liposuction.

**Bone health.** Loss of bone mineral density (BMD) with ADT for prostate cancer is well recognized, with significant loss within 12 months of starting therapy; the annual loss is 2–8% per year at the lumbar spine and 2–6% at the hip. The loss appears to continue indefinitely while treatment continues, and there is no recovery after therapy ceases. Just under 20% of men surviving at least 5 years after a diagnosis of prostate cancer have a fracture if treated with ADT, compared with about 13% of men who do not receive this therapy; this is equivalent to one additional fracture for every 28 men treated with ADT.

Vitamin D deficiency exacerbates the development of osteoporosis, so vitamin D status should be evaluated and corrected before starting ADT.

Bisphosphonates (zoledronic acid [zoledronate], pamidronic acid [pamidronate] and alendronic acid [alendronate]) have been shown to prevent bone loss in prospective studies in men receiving ADT, and increased BMD in one randomized controlled trial.

Bisphosphonates and the anti-RANKL monoclonal antibody denosumab (see pages 113–14) have also been shown to reduce the incidence of skeletal-related events in men with prostate cancer. Further prospective trials are required to assess the efficacy and cost-effectiveness of bisphosphonates in men with prostate cancer who require ADT. Until the results from these trials become available, suggestions for the management of bone effects in men receiving ADT include baseline and yearly measurements of BMD. Baseline calcium, phosphate, liver function, thyroid function, 25-hydroxy vitamin D and parathyroid hormone should be measured, and calcium and vitamin D supplementation as well as isometric exercises, should be encouraged. Osteonecrosis of the jaw is a rare complication of bisphosphonate therapy.

**Metabolic syndrome and cardiovascular risk.** Metabolic syndrome is a constellation of cardiovascular risk factors (e.g. fasting hyperglycemia, hypertriglyceridemia, decreased serum high-density lipoprotein [HDL] cholesterol, increases in waist circumference and waist to hip ratio, and hypertension) that have been reported to be increased in men receiving ADT.

The first study to report an increase in cardiovascular risk in men treated with ADT was a retrospective study of 79 196 men in whom an increased risk of coronary disease, myocardial infarction and ventricular arrhythmia was identified. Another large retrospective study also suggested a 20% increase in cardiovascular morbidity with 1 year of ADT. A study by D'Amico et al. reported that, in men over 65 years, treatment with ADT decreased the time to fatal myocardial infarction compared with men not receiving this therapy. However, a large number of other studies have not shown any major differences in cardiovascular morbidity.

As this area is controversial, it is prudent to critically weigh the risks and benefits of ADT in men with cardiovascular risk factors. It is also important to monitor all the risk factors in all men undergoing ADT, and to treat these risk factors where appropriate.

*Lipid profile.* ADT alters lipid profiles, potentially increasing cardiovascular risk. Total cholesterol rises by approximately 10%, triglycerides by 25% and low-density lipoprotein (LDL)-cholesterol by 7%. However, this may be counteracted by a reported 11% rise in HDL-cholesterol levels.

*Insulin sensitivity* is related to testosterone levels; ADT reduces insulin sensitivity. A number of large studies have reported a 19–49% increase in the risk of developing diabetes in men receiving ADT.

*Waist circumference* increases while on ADT, but increased waist to hip ratio and hypertension have not been consistently reported in trials.

*Management.* A detailed medical examination and history should be taken before ADT is started, with particular focus on cardiovascular risk factors. This will enable proactive management before any condition becomes worse as a consequence of ADT.

Bodyweight, blood pressure, serum lipids and fasting blood glucose should be monitored regularly during ADT (at 3-monthly intervals).

Patients at risk should be advised to make lifestyle changes before and while using ADT: stop smoking, lose weight if necessary, increase physical activity, eat a healthy diet.

Individual risk factors should be actively managed – for example, lipid-lowering agents for hyperlipidemia and glucose-lowering agents for diabetes.

---

**Key points – survivorship and treatment complications**

- Men with prostate cancer require emotional support as well as information on probable outcomes and the effects of the disease and its treatment.
- Sexual dysfunction is a common sequela of prostate cancer treatment. An open and informed discussion with the patient and his partner will do much to counter anxiety and loss of self-esteem.
- Erectile dysfunction can often be improved with phosphodiesterase-5 (PDE5) inhibitors, prostaglandin suppositories or injections, or mechanical vacuum devices.
- Loss of libido can be reduced by using antiandrogens to treat prostate cancer in preference to bilateral orchidectomy or a luteinizing hormone-releasing hormone (LHRH) analog/ antagonist.
- Osteoporosis and fractures are side effects of long-term androgen deprivation therapy (ADT): vitamin D status should be evaluated before starting ADT, and calcium and vitamin D supplementation, as well as isometric exercises, encouraged during treatment.
- It is prudent to weigh the risks and benefits of ADT in men with cardiovascular risk factors and to monitor all risk factors during therapy. At-risk patients should be advised to make lifestyle changes as appropriate (e.g. stop smoking, lose weight, increase physical activity, improve diet).

## Key references

Alibhai SM, Duong-Hua M, Sutradhar R et al. Impact of androgen deprivation therapy on cardiovascular disease and diabetes. *J Clin Oncol* 2009;27:3452–8.

Carson C, McMahon CG. *Fast Facts: Erectile Dysfunction*, 4th edn. Oxford: Health Press Ltd, 2008.

D'Amico AV, Denham JW, Crook J et al. Influence of androgen suppression therapy for prostate cancer on the frequency and timing of fatal myocardial infarctions. *J Clin Oncol* 2007;25:2420–5.

Holmes-Walker DJ, Woo H, Gurney H et al. Maintaining bone health in patients with prostate cancer. *Med J Aust* 2006;184:176–9.

Levine GN, D'Amico AV, Berger P et al. Androgen-deprivation therapy in prostate cancer and cardiovascular risk: a science advisory from the American Heart Association, American Cancer Society, and American Urological Association: endorsed by the American Society for Radiation Oncology. *Circulation* 2010;121:833–40.

Montorsi F, Guazzoni G, Strambi LF et al. Recovery of spontaneous erectile function after nerve-sparing radical retropubic prostatectomy with and without early intracavernous injections of alprostadil: results of a prospective, randomized trial. *J Urol* 1997;58:1408–10.

Montorsi F, Nathan HP, McCullough A et al. Tadalafil in the treatment of erectile dysfunction following bilateral nerve sparing radical retropubic prostatectomy: a randomized, double-blind, placebo controlled trial. *J Urol* 2004;172:1036–41.

Penson DF, McLerran D, Feng Z et al. 5-year urinary and sexual outcomes after radical prostatectomy: results from the Prostate Cancer Outcomes Study. *J Urol* 2008;179(suppl):S40–4.

Saad F, Adachi JD, Brown JP et al. Cancer treatment-induced bone loss in breast and prostate cancer. *J Clin Oncol* 2008;26:5465–76.

Saigal CS, Gore JL, Krupski TL et al. Androgen deprivation therapy increases cardiovascular morbidity in men with prostate cancer. *Cancer* 2007;110:1493–500.

Scher HI, Fizazi K, Saad F et al. Increased survival with enzalutamide in prostate cancer after chemotherapy. *N Engl J Med* 2012;367:1187–97.

Slack A, Newman DK, Wein AJ. *Fast Facts: Bladder Disorders*, 2nd edn. Oxford: Health Press Ltd, 2011.

Smith MR, Finkelstein JS, McGovern FJ et al. Changes in body composition during androgen deprivation therapy for prostate cancer. *J Clin Endocrinol Metab* 2002;87:599–603.

Smith MR, Lee H, McGovern F et al. Metabolic changes during gonadotropin-releasing hormone agonist therapy for prostate cancer: differences from the classic metabolic syndrome. *Cancer* 2008;112:2188–94.

Smith MR, Lee H, Nathan DM. Insulin sensitivity during combined androgen blockade for prostate cancer. *J Clin Endocrinol Metab* 2006;91:1305–8.

# Useful resources

## UK

**Cancer Research UK**
Tel: +44 (0)20 7242 0200
www.cancerresearchuk.org

**Macmillan Cancer Support**
Helpline: 0808 808 00 00
www.macmillan.org.uk

**Marie Curie Cancer Care**
Patient referrals: 0845 056 7899
www.mariecurie.org.uk

**Men's Health Forum**
Tel: +44 (0)20 7922 7908
www.menshealthforum.org.uk

**Prostate Cancer Research Centre**
www.prostate-cancer-research.org.uk

**Prostate Cancer UK**
Helpline: 0800 074 8383
www.prostatecanceruk.org

**The Urology Foundation**
www.theurologyfoundation.org
Tel: +44 (0)20 7713 9538

## USA

**American Cancer Society**
Toll-free: 1 800 227 2345
www.cancer.org

**American Urological Association**
Toll-free: 1 866 746 4282
Tel: +1 410 689 3700
www.auanet.org

**National Cancer Institute**
Toll-free: 1 800 422 6237
www.cancer.gov/cancertopics/types/
prostate

**Prostate Cancer Foundation**
Tel: +1 310 570 4700
Toll-free: 1 800 757 2873
www.pcf.org

**Prostate Cancer Research Institute**
Tel: +1 310 743 2116
Helpline: 1 800 641 7274
www.prostate-cancer.org

**Prostate Conditions Education Council**
Tel: +1 303 316 4685
Toll-free: 1 866 477 6788
www.prostateconditions.org

**ZERO – The End of Prostate Cancer**
Tel: +1 202 463 9455
Toll-free: 1 888 245 9455
www.zerocancer.org

**International**

European Association of Urology

Tel: + 31 (0)26 389 06 80

info@uroweb.org

www.uroweb.org

Prostate Cancer Canada

Tel: +1 416 441 2131

Toll-free: 1 888 255 0333

www.prostatecancer.ca

Prostate Cancer Foundation of Australia

Tel: +61 (0)2 9438 7000

Toll-free: 1800 220 099

www.prostate.org.au

Prostate Cancer Foundation of South Africa

Tel: +27 (0)11 791 1791

www.prostatecancerfoundation.co.za

**Other useful websites**

Embarrassing Problems

www.embarrassingproblems.com

Hormone-Refractory Prostate Cancer

www.hrpca.org

James Buchanan Brady Urological Institute

urology.jhu.edu

Johns Hopkins Medicine

www.hopkinsmedicine.org

Mayo Clinic prostate cancer

www.mayoclinic.com/health/prostate-cancer/DS00043

Memorial Sloan-Kettering Cancer Center

www.mskcc.org

Patient Pictures

www.patientpictures.com/urology

William Catalona

(developer of the PSA test)
www.drcatalona.com

---

# *FastTest*

## You've read the book ... now test yourself with key questions from the authors

- Go to the FastTest for this title
  *FREE* at fastfacts.com

- Approximate time **10 minutes**

- For best retention of the key issues, try taking the FastTest before and after reading

# Index

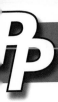
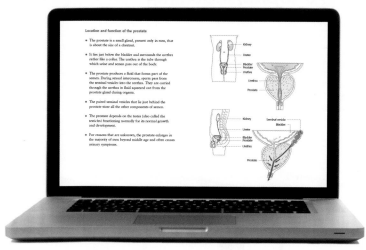

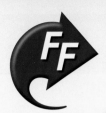
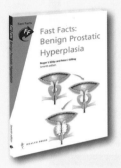
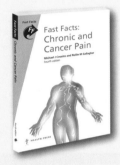
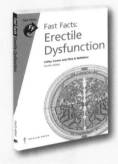
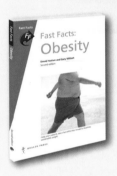
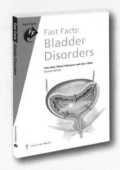
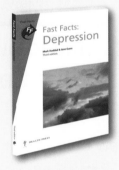
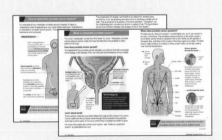
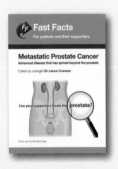